# Legal and Ethical Issues: To Know, To Reason, To Act

*Guest Editors*

DANA BJARNASON, PhD, RN, NE-BC
MICHELE A. CARTER, PhD

# NURSING CLINICS
# OF NORTH AMERICA

www.nursing.theclinics.com

*Consulting Editor*
SUZANNE S. PREVOST, RN, PhD, COI

December 2009 • Volume 44 • Number 4

SAUNDERS an imprint of ELSEVIER, Inc.

## W.B. SAUNDERS COMPANY

*A Division of Elsevier Inc.*

1600 John F. Kennedy Blvd., Suite 1800 • Philadelphia, PA 19103-2899

http://www.theclinics.com

**NURSING CLINICS OF NORTH AMERICA Volume 44, Number 4**
**December 2009 ISSN 0029-6465, ISBN-13: 978-1-4377-1246-9, ISBN-10: 1-4377-1246-0**

Editor: Katie Hartner
Developmental Editor: Donald Mumford

*Nursing Clinics of North America* (ISSN 0029-6465) is published quarterly by Elsevier Inc., 360 Park Avenue South, New York, NY 10010-1710. Months of issue are March, June, September, and December. Periodicals postage paid at New York, NY and additional mailing offices. Subscription price per year is, $133.00 (US individuals), $306.00 (US institutions), $228.00 (international individuals), $374.00 (international institutions), $184.00 (Canadian individuals), $374.00 (Canadian institutions), $70.00 (US students), and $115.00 (international students). To receive student/resident rate, orders must be accompanied by name of affiliated institution, date of term, and the signature of program/residency coordinator on institution letterhead. Orders will be billed at individual rate until proof of status is received. Foreign air speed delivery is included in all *Clinics* subscription prices. All prices are subject to change without notice. **POSTMASTER:** Send address changes to *Nursing Clinics*, Elsevier Health Sciences Division, Subscription Customer Service, 3251 Riverport Lane, Maryland Heights, MO 63043. **Customer Service: Telephone:1-800-654-2452 (U.S. and Canada); 1-314-447-8871 (outside U.S. and Canada). Fax: 1-314-447-8029. E-mail: JournalsCustomerService-usa@elsevier.com** (for print support) and **JournalsOnlineSupport-usa@elsevier.com** (for online support).

*Nursing Clinics of North America* is covered in *EMBASE/Excerpta Medica, MEDLINE/PubMed (Index Medicus), Social Sciences Citation Index, Current Contents, ASCA, Cumulative Index to Nursing, RNdex Top 100,* and Allied Health Literature and International Nursing Index (INI).

Printed in the United States of America.

# Contributors

## CONSULTING EDITOR

**SUZANNE S. PREVOST, RN, PhD, COI**
Associate Dean, Practice and Community Engagement, University of Kentucky, Lexington, Kentucky

## GUEST EDITORS

**DANA BJARNASON, PhD, RN, NE-BC**
Associate Administrator and Chief Nursing Officer, Ben Taub General Hospital; and Quentin Mease Community Hospital, Houston, Texas

**MICHELE A. CARTER, PhD**
Frances C. and Courtney M. Townsend, Sr, MD Professor in Medical Ethics; Associate Professor, Institute for the Medical Humanities, Department of Preventive Medicine and Community Health; and Director, UTMB Ethics Consultation Services, The University of Texas Medical Branch, University Boulevard, Galveston, Texas

## AUTHORS

**DANA BJARNASON, PhD, RN, NE-BC**
Associate Administrator and Chief Nursing Officer, Ben Taub General Hospital; and Quentin Mease Community Hospital, Houston, Texas

**MICHELE A. CARTER, PhD**
Frances C. and Courtney M. Townsend, Sr, MD Professor in Medical Ethics; Associate Professor, Institute for the Medical Humanities, Department of Preventive Medicine and Community Health; and Director, UTMB Ethics Consultation Services, The University of Texas Medical Branch, University Boulevard, Galveston, Texas

**ELIZABETH CLOYD, MBA, RN, NEA-BC, FACHE**
Executive Vice President and Chief Nurse Executive, Harris County Hospital District, Houston, Texas

**ERNESTINE (Tina) CUELLAR, RN, PhD**
Assistant Professor and Associate Dean for Student Affairs, University of Texas Medical Branch, School of Nursing, University Boulevard, Galveston; Lt. Colonel, United States Air Force Reserve, North Carolina; and Chief, Mental Health Department, 433rd Aeromedical Staging Squadron, Lackland Air Force Base, San Antonio, Texas

**MAUREEN EDGERLY, RN, MA**
Senior Research Nurse Specialist, National Cancer Institute, Medical Oncology Branch, Bethesda, Maryland

**CHRISTINE GRADY, RN, PhD**
Acting Chief, Department of Bioethics, National Institutes of Health Clinical Center, Bethesda, Maryland

**REBEKAH HAMILTON, PhD, RN**
Assistant Professor, Department of Women, Children and Family Health Science (MC 802), College of Nursing, University of Illinois at Chicago, Chicago, Illinois

**KEVIN HOOK, MA, MSN, CRNP**
Coordinator, Advanced Practice Nursing and Ethics Integration, Golden Living Centers, Westmont, New Jersey

**KAREN ISEMINGER, PhD, FNP**
Director of Ethics Integration, St. Vincent Health, Indianapolis, Indiana

**TAYRAY JASMINE, PhD, MSN, RN**
Director of Operational Support, Harris County Hospital District, Harris County, Houston; and Healthcare Consultant, Collective Healthcare Services, Pearland, Texas

**LISA KIRK, RN, BSN, CWOCN**
Wound, Ostomy, Continence Nurse, Clarian Health Partners, Riley Hospital for Children, Indianapolis, Indiana

**CYNTHIA ANN LaSALA, MS, RN**
Clinical Nurse Specialist, Medicine and Oncology, Massachusetts General Hospital, Boston, Massachusetts; and Member, American Nurses Association Center for Ethics and Human Rights Advisory Board, Silver Spring, Maryland

**FRANCESCA LEVITT, MSN, RN-BC, CNS**
Surgical Clinical Nurse Specialist, St. Vincent Hospital, Indianapolis, Indiana

**LEIGH ANN McINNIS, PhD, RN, FNP-BC**
Associate Professor of Nursing; Associate Director Online Programs, Middle Tennessee State University, School of Nursing; and Family Nurse Practitioner, Rutherford County Primary Care and Hope Clinic, Murfreesboro, Tennessee

**JoANN MICK, PhD, RN, AOCN, NEA-BC**
Director, Nursing Research and Clinical Outcomes, Harris County Hospital District, Houston, Texas

**CHERYL MONTURO, PhD, MBE, CRNP**
Assistant Professor of Nursing and John A. Harford Foundation Claire M. Fagin Fellow, West Chester University College of Health Sciences, Department of Nursing, West Chester, Pennsylvania

**LYNN C. PARSONS, DSN, RN, CNA-BC**
Professor and Director, Middle Tennessee State University, School of Nursing, Murfreesboro, Tennessee

**JULIA A. THOMPSON, PhD, RN, CIP**
Administrative Director, Research and Sponsored Programs, Harris County Hospital District, Houston, Texas

**CHERYL ELLIS VAIANI, PhD**
Assistant Professor, Institute for the Medical Humanities, Department of Preventative Medicine and Community Health and Clinical Ethicist, Institutional Ethics Program, University of Texas Medical Branch, Galveston, Texas

# Contents

> This article uses philosophical inquiry to present the relationship between the helping role in nursing and the concept of trust essential to it. It characterizes helping as the moral center of the nurse-patient relationship and discusses how patients' expectations of help and caring create obligations of trustworthiness on the part of the nurse. It uses literature from various disciplines to examine different theoretical accounts of trust, each presenting important features of trust relationships that apply to health care professionals, patients, and families. Exploring the concept of trust, and the key leverage points that elicit it, develops a thesis that nurses can improve their understanding of the principal attributes and the conditions that foster or impede trust. The article concludes that trust is the core moral ingredient of helping relationships. Trust as a moral value is even more basic than duties of beneficence, respect, veracity, and autonomy. Trust is the confident expectation that others can be relied upon to act with good will and to secure what is best for the person seeking help.

> The moral practice of nursing requires the difficult work of discerning the best response to an ethical quandary. Determining the right course of action can rarely be discovered by assuming that one value, one theory, one point of view will always and reliably identify the morality of an action. Thus, the role of a nurse is an inherently moral activity that is at the heart and soul of health care. Practitioners who move too quickly to a state of moral certainty about a decision may be missing essential components of the enactment of moral agency. Personal integrity and professional integrity, patient interests, society's expectation of a profession, the balance between rights and obligations within the nurse-patient relationship, acting according to one's conscience, power, control, and moral certainty are a few of the topics that enrich thinking about the moral richness of nursing practice, and will encourage readers to know, to reason, and to act in ways that demonstrate reflective moral judgment.

> Nursing is widely considered as an art and a science, wherein caring forms the theoretical framework of nursing. Nursing and caring are grounded in

a relational understanding, unity, and connection between the professional nurse and the patient. Task-oriented approaches challenge nurses in keeping care in nursing. This challenge is ongoing as professional nurses strive to maintain the concept, art, and act of caring as the moral center of the nursing profession. Keeping the care in nursing involves the application of art and science through theoretical concepts, scientific research, conscious commitment to the art of caring as an identity of nursing, and purposeful efforts to include caring behaviors during each nurse-patient interaction. This article discusses the profession of nursing as an art and a science, and it explores the challenges associated with keeping the care in nursing.

The therapeutic nature of the nurse-patient relationship is grounded in an ethic of caring. Florence Nightingale envisioned nursing as an art and a science…a blending of humanistic, caring presence with evidence-based knowledge and exquisite skill. In this article, the author explores the caring practice of nursing as a framework for understanding moral accountability and integrity in practice. Being morally accountable and responsible for one's judgment and actions is central to the nurse's role as a moral agent. Nurses who practice with moral integrity possess a strong sense of themselves and act in ways consistent with what they understand is the right thing to do. A review of the literature related to caring theory, the concepts of moral accountability and integrity, and the documents that speak of these values and concepts in professional practice (eg, *Code of Ethics for Nurses with Interpretive Statements*, *Nursing's Social Policy Statement*) are presented in this article.

The Human Genome Project will change how health is defined and how disease is prevented, diagnosed, and treated. As the largest group of health care providers in contact with patients, nurses need to be competent in the science of genetics. Beyond this, nurses need to understand the complexities that arise in genomic health care. Ethical, legal, and social issues are integral to the delivery of genomic health care, and nurses must have an astute understanding of such complexities. What it means to know, to reason, and to act in this postgenomic age is explored.

This article addresses nursing presence, a phenomenon essential to holistic nursing care. The concept is introduced and explained, supporting background information is reviewed, barriers are identified, and successful applications are illustrated in different clinical settings. Avowing that metaphysical knowledge is the underpinning to the art of nursing presence, a Transformative Nursing Presence Model is offered as a distinctive framework for nurses and organizations interested in fostering enhanced nursing presence.

This article discusses delegation challenges and legal and regulatory oversight associated with delegation in the clinical practice setting. The authors address moral and legal attributes of the roles and responsibilities of health care providers regarding delegating health care interventions. The article also explores guiding principles and rules of delegation within professional standards, national practice guidelines, and state nurse practice acts. Nurse experts provide thoughtful reflection on nursing models and the role of delegation, emphasizing the critical role of delegation in extending the role of the health care professional in patient care services.

Clinical research is a systematic investigation of human biology, health, or illness involving human beings. It builds on laboratory and animal studies and often involves clinical trials, which are specifically designed to test the safety and efficacy of interventions in humans. Nurses are critical to the conduct of ethical clinical research and face clinical, ethical, and regulatory challenges in research in many diverse roles. Understanding and addressing the ethical challenges that complicate clinical research is integral to upholding the moral commitment that nurses make to patients, including protecting their rights and ensuring their safety as patients and as research participants.

During the past century, nurses have served as caregivers for United States military personnel in every major theater of war. Military nurses in the war zone deliver patient care while working in austere conditions, and are under constant threat of personal danger. This article gives a historical overview of the role of nurses in war zones, followed by a review from the perspectives of environment, safety, the nature of injuries, and treatment of military personnel and civilians.

Culture has been defined as the thoughts, communications, actions, customs, beliefs, values, and institutions of racial, ethnic, religious, or social groups. A culture of nursing refers to the learned and transmitted lifeways, values, symbols, patterns, and normative practices of members of the nursing profession of a particular society. To serve the unique and diverse needs of patients in the United States, it is imperative that nurses understand the importance of cultural differences by valuing, incorporating, and examining their own health-related values and beliefs and those of their health care organizations, for only then can they support the principle of respect for persons and the ideal of transcultural care.

The withdrawal, withholding, or implementation of life-sustaining treatments such as artificial nutrition and hydration challenge nurses on a daily basis. To meet these challenges, nurses need the composite skills of moral and ethical discernment, practical wisdom and a knowledge base that justifies reasoning and actions that support patient and family decision making. Nurses' moral knowledge develops through experiential learning, didactic learning, and deliberation of ethical principles that merge with moral intuition, ethical codes, and moral theories. Only when a nurse becomes skilled and confident in gathering empiric and ethical knowledge can he or she fully act as a moral agent in assisting families faced with making highly emotional decisions regarding the provision, withholding, or withdrawal of artificial nutrition and hydration.

The influence of religious beliefs and practices at the end of life is under-investigated. Given nursing's advocacy role and the intimate and personal nature of the dimensions of religiosity and the end of life, exploring the multidimensional interplay of religiosity and end-of-life care is a significant aspect of the nurse-patient relationship and must be better understood. The question that must be faced is whether nurses' own belief systems impinge on or influence patient care, especially for patients who are at the end of life. When nurses understand their own beliefs and respect the religious practices and needs of patients and their families, it deepens the humanistic dimensions of the nurse-patient relationship.

## THE CLINICS ARE NOW AVAILABLE ONLINE!

Access your subscription at:
**www.theclinics.com**

# Preface
# To Know, To Reason, To Act

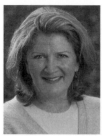 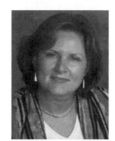

Dana Bjarnason, PhD, RN, NE-BC    Michele A. Carter, PhD
*Guest Editors*

Ethics is fundamentally an inquiry into human experience and the values, beliefs, and judgments that guide human action. Ethical inquiry and reflection in nursing are concerned with critically examining which values, actions, or standards ought to govern our personal and professional lives as well as our relationships with others. This examination ranges over a wide territory of concerns and aspirations, many of which are reflected in historical traditions, contemporary practice guidelines, and ageless quests regarding the good life and what it means to be a person of good character. An understanding of the core ethical values and virtues that embody the nursing profession is an essential component of responsible knowing, ethical discernment, and moral agency. This understanding in turn helps build allegiance to a professional ethos whereby special commitments and duties to others are rightly expected, honored, and justified. Understanding these expectations and acting on behalf of the promises they embody help define and shape the personal integrity of the nurse and the social character of the profession itself.

Ethical inquiry and reflection in nursing are also about moral conflict and the choices we are called upon to make and defend. As a humanistic and altruistic endeavor, nursing is an art as well as a science, a philosophy as well as a practice. In this issue of *Nursing Clinics of North America*, we develop the themes of nursing knowledge, nursing reason, and nursing action around a diverse set of moral concerns and problems in contemporary practice settings. Although these settings encompass an increasing diversity of venues in nursing education, scholarship, research, and clinical practice, the enduring subject of each inquiry is always the person whose illness, disease, injury, or defeat makes possible the moral activity of nursing. Integrating the themes of knowing, reasoning, and acting into a diverse set of inquiries and reflections by nurse writers from a variety of disciplines provides a unique opportunity to enhance appreciation for the moral dimensions of nursing.

Embodying the trust imparted upon nurses by patients demands embracing moral and humanistic ideals. The very essence of nursing—knowing, reasoning, and acting

doi:10.1016/j.cnur.2009.09.001
0029-6465/09/$ – see front matter © 2009 Elsevier Inc. All rights reserved.

on behalf of people, in sickness or in health—is enhanced by knowledge and insights derived not only from nursing, but also acquired from interdisciplinary domains. These forms of knowledge and the ability to appropriately apply them in the lives of patients constitute the core foundation of nursing as a helping profession.

As nursing continues to deepen its commitment to the ideals embedded in its social contract, new forms of practice and critical reflection emerge. Each of the authors whose work is presented here offers a unique perspective on the nature of nursing, with special emphasis on issues involving legal and ethical norms. Although these nurses are employed in a variety of health care settings and contexts, each with its own set of concerns and opportunities, they share a common passion for scholarly reflection, the courage to act on their moral convictions, and the belief that the authentic character of nursing resides in nurses themselves.

Dana Bjarnason, PhD, RN, NE-BC
Ben Taub General Hospital
1504 Taub Loop
Houston, TX 77030

Michele A. Carter, PhD
Institute for the Medical Humanities
Department of Preventive Medicine and Community Health
UTMB Ethics Consultation Services
The University of Texas Medical Branch
301 University Boulevard
Galveston, Texas 77555–1311

E-mail addresses:
dana_bjarnason@hchd.tmc.edu (D. Bjarnason)
mcarter@utmb.edu (M.A. Carter)

# Trust, Power, and Vulnerability: A Discourse on Helping in Nursing

Michele A. Carter, PhD

KEYWORDS

• Trust • Power • Vulnerability • Morality • Ethical responsibility

## THE HELPING ROLE IN NURSING

Nursing has long considered its practice in humanistic terms, a deliberate blend of knowledge, agency, reasoning, and action in the service of others. Illness, and the threat of pain, suffering, loss, and/or death are unavoidable conditions of human life. The experience of illness often provokes feelings of vulnerability, not only in patients but for those who witness their loss and attempt to care for them. When ill, patients depend on the technical knowledge and professional skills of the provider, often a previously unfamiliar individual, in order to regain health, functional status, and well-being. Additionally, patients depend on providers to help, to be worthy of trust, to respond morally to their suffering and vulnerabilities, and to provide ethically sensitive care in wide variety of practice settings and situations. This dependence creates unique ethical responsibilities in terms of the helping role and the forms of care embedded in it.

Helping is integral to clinical nursing and has been defined as "any action that enables the individual to overcome whatever interferes with his ability to function capably in relation to his situation."[1] When patients experience a need for help and when nurses initiate the process of assisting patients to sustain themselves through illness and toward health or wholeness, a therapeutic relationship is born. The nurse-patient relationship is regarded by nurses as "a sacred, privileged trust" and the cornerstone of professional nursing practice.[2] This relationship—the foundation of clinical practice and the common bond between the nurse and patient—demarcates the practitioner's field of knowledge and legitimizes various personal and private interventions and actions for which nurses are held accountable. It operates in various domains but essentially comprises 4 necessary components: (1) the patient in need of

Institute for the Medical Humanities, Department of Preventive Medicine and Community Health, UTMB Ethics Consultation Services, The University of Texas Medical Branch, 301 University Boulevard, Galveston, TX 77555-1311, USA
*E-mail address:* mcarter@utmb.edu

Nurs Clin N Am 44 (2009) 393–405
doi:10.1016/j.cnur.2009.07.012
0029-6465/09/$ – see front matter © 2009 Elsevier Inc. All rights reserved.

assistance, (2) the nurse professional who provides help, (3) a societal context for the delivery of needed services, including other members of the health care team, and (4) the diverse and sometimes competing conceptualizations about health, illness, caring, coping, and healing. Insofar as the nurse-patient relationship is an interpersonal process in which both parties have an emotional involvement with each other, there is a degree of mutuality and reciprocity whereby needs and expectations are shared. Relationships that operate as generalized exchanges between people operate from a mode of trust or faith—there is an expectation that one who helps will be helped in return, even if by different persons.[3] This reciprocity is the genesis of the nursing process and the means of exchanging therapeutic communication strategies that reflect caring interactions.

By virtue of their specialized knowledge, skills, and expertise, nurses assume the role of helper and bear the responsibility of fulfilling the duties and responsibilities of the helper role, as facilitator, advocate, coordinator, counselor, or caregiver. Patients, made vulnerable by the experience of illness and the need to depend on others, contribute their own unique characteristics, skills, and abilities to the relationship. The nurse-patient encounter is therapeutic in nature, because it is aimed at the patient's expressed or implicit desire for change. When a patient is unable to perform activities of daily living or, independently, of self-care, the helping role takes on specific characteristics of caregiving. Here, helping may involve various discrete forms of caring, such as assisting the patient in learning to live with chronic ailments or permanent loss of function, relating to the individual in pain, and validating the individual's experience of loneliness or grief, the dislocation of self in the diseases of addiction, and the existential crises in meaning at the end of life. Knowledge-based caring behavior is expressed in these encounters, and the relationship thus becomes the moral center of nursing.

## TRUST AND HELPING RELATIONSHIPS

Many nurse scholars have proposed various models of the different phases in the formation of helping relationships and the dynamic interchange of knowledge, attitudes, and skills occurring in them.[4] Most of these models make the assumption that trust is an important consideration in the helping relationship and seem to assume that it can be readily established. It is not clear that trust can simply be assumed, although the human need for relatedness and connection creates the desire to trust, and therapeutic relationships have better outcomes when trust formation has been made possible and morally legitimate. Nurses know that the trust they need to be effective will be lost if they fail to meet the expectations of patients; yet, although the needs and interests of each patient are different, and the ability and capacity of each nurse to meet those needs can vary, trust can be a risky venture.

Many nursing scholars theorize that the helping role requires the nurse to develop competencies in creating a healing environment for patients and in being present as they respond to the unique needs of patients. Indeed, Florence Nightingale argues that it is the nurse's core responsibility to use the tools of science "as they further the healing mission."[5] In using the tools of nursing knowledge to further the health-related aspirations of a patient, nurses are expected to reason about a wide range of human needs and vulnerabilities and to act responsibly on them. These expectations form the basis of trusting behavior and claims made on behalf of it. Inherent to the nurse-patient relationship are specific role-related norms, competencies, and obligations, pertaining to the interpersonal transactions within the relationship and to the increasingly complex social systems in which nursing is practiced and taught. The concept of trust, applicable to helping relationships, incorporates interpersonal relations and institutional systems, as discussed in the following section. Because the relationships formed between patients and nurses are uniquely asymmetrical in knowledge, dependence, and vulnerability, responsible helping includes consideration of the manner in which a nurse uses the legitimate power of the professional role.

## WHAT IS TRUST?

Trust is most often a "given" in social life. Many of the helping professions make explicit claims regarding the value and necessity of trust. Trust is a feature of everyday life, but its meaning can be explored from various perspectives, each providing conceptual distinctions that are relevant for the claims made on its behalf. In assessing its utility as a concept deserving of scientific application, trust has been found to be an ambiguous construct in need of more mature exploration.[6] Despite the expressed importance it holds in issues of healing, compliance, and patient satisfaction, the concept of trust has not been adequately analyzed nor demarcated from closely related constructs, such as reliance, confidence, and faith. Until recently, there has been a surprising lack of scholarship in the nursing literature on the nature of interpersonal trust, the features which characterize trusting behavior, the manner in which trust develops, or the conditions on which trust is based.

In addition, the essential attributes of trust as a moral value have not received appropriate attention in the nursing literature or in applied ethics. Many profound and provocative questions have simply not been raised. Is it sensible, or rational, or moral, for patients to simply obey a nonevidentiary imperative to trust their health care professionals? Should patients obey their physicians without evaluating the grounds of their medical advice? Should patients remain confident that their best interests can be better ascertained by their nurses than by themselves, as autonomous agents exhibiting their rights to self-determination? Given the empirical evidence of the rising incidence of abuses of trust in government and other institutions in the United States over the past 30 years,[7] what accounts for these abuses and what harm is done to trust? Furthermore, what do patients lose when trust is damaged by these abuses and how does this betrayal affect the practitioner's claims for trustworthiness? Although the need for trust in others and in health care organizations is necessary, given the increasingly complex and competitive global marketplace, the frequent invocations to trust seem weak without any conceptual analysis of the essential elements of trust as a social and ethical value. The concept of trust deserves more rigorous attention, because of its significance to nursing and to future patients who are recipients of nursing's professional services.

One of the paradoxes of trust is that trust never grows without our taking the risk of placing our trust in others. This has important implications in the forming and fostering of trust in professional-patient relationships and in the health care system itself. Approaching the concept of trust as an interpersonal good and an element of professional accountability illustrates the complexities involved in understanding how it can be offered, earned, and sustained. In the discussion that follows, the concept of trust is analyzed from various disciplinary perspectives, which embody important insights that contribute to professional nursing practice.

## PHILOSOPHICAL APPROACHES

Sissela Bok[8] is one of the first philosophers to address the ethics of trust fairly directly. She states that "[w]hatever matters to human beings, trust is the atmosphere in which it thrives." According to Bok, trust is a social good to be protected as much as the air we breathe and the water we drink. "When it is damaged, the community as a whole suffers; and when it is destroyed, societies falter and collapse." She lists 3 different kinds of trust: (1) that you will treat me fairly, (2) that you will have my interests at heart, and (3) that you will do me no harm. She asks whether one could ever have any one of these kinds of trust if one did not have a genuine confidence in the truthfulness of others. She questions whether, without such confidence in the word of others, there is any way to assess their fairness or their intentions to help or to harm. Bok's analysis of trust establishes an important ingredient: that trust is based on perceptions of consistency in the words and actions of others. The forms of trust she discusses have relevance for the therapeutic relationship, because they reflect the moral principles of justice, beneficence, and nonmaleficence, each embodying expectations inherent in the professional practice of nursing. Bok does not provide a definition of trust or attempt to discern its conceptual demarcation from related concepts, such a reliance or confidence; however, by linking the attitude of trust with rhetorical claims of honesty and consistency, she captures an important aspect of trustworthiness in professional life. In fact, in a Gallup poll surveying public views on the "honesty and ethical standards" of members of 21 different professions, nurses continued to have top ranking, with 84% of Americans rating their honesty or ethical standards as "high" or "very high."[9] Empirical claims of this sort help generate expectations and invocations regarding the values and virtues associated with trust, but they fail to describe the nature of trust relations or the conditions that nourish or erode them. In addition to honesty and compliance with ethical standards, nurses make commitments to help individuals in achieving health-related goals, in ways that also sustain their own values, rights, and responsibilities. Therefore, although honesty, including avoiding deception, is part of trustworthiness in others, trust entails more than this simple account.

The search for such an account of trust relationships has recently been undertaken by philosopher Annette Baier.[10,11] Baier claims that morality itself requires trust to thrive and that morality must take into account the vulnerability of persons who are in unequal relationships of power to one another. She is interested in the question of how we should judge trust relationships from a moral point of view and is concerned with the problem of exploitation that arises in relationships of unequal power.

On her highly influential account, trust is often a mixture of reliance, confidence, and dependence. Reliance is an attitude toward another person's competence to perform certain acts or to have certain dependable habits. Reliance on others to perform their work competently, may be compatible with various motivations, but essentially, we expect people to act in certain ways because they are required to do so. For example, when relying on someone to show up to an appointment, one is depending on the person to do so, but this type of reliance is not a form of trusting per se. If that person fails to be reliable, the response may be one of disappointment, but not betrayal. Trust, according to Baier, means depending on another's good will. In depending on someone's good will, there is a degree of confidence that the person will not take advantage of this dependence or show indifference, but there is always the possibility of betrayal. One is vulnerable in that the dependence on that good will may be limited or misused, and thus, one is open to the possibility of risk. Hence, trust is an "accepted vulnerability to another's possible but not expected ill will (or lack of good will) toward one."[11] As such, trust implies confidence or reliance on one's agreement. Presumably, "good will" refers to caring about the good of others and being concerned for their welfare. Baier goes on to say that furthering the good of others requires a type of considered judgment. Trust is reasonable insofar as it is based on either good grounds for such confidence in another's good will or the absence of good grounds for expecting their ill will or perhaps, their indifference. Trust, at least between articulate adults, can thus be characterized as reliance on others' competency and willingness to look after the things that one cares about, which are entrusted to their care, rather than to harm them.

Additionally, Baier claims that what people typically value (presumably health and well-being are likely candidates) are things that cannot be single-handedly created or sustained. Consequently, people get into positions where they can injure others if they choose. She bases this claim on the assumption that nobody is entirely self-sufficient and, therefore, one must entrust to others the care of things that one cares about. Inherently, people trust that others will not use their power in ways that undermine the things cared about or that inflict some other possible harm. In Baier's view, trust is letting other persons take care of something that the truster cares about, wherein such "caring" involves some exercise of discretionary powers. In applying this account of trust to the practitioner-patient relationship, furthering the patient's good requires that professionals use their discretion to decide how best to serve the interests of patients. When patients allow their practitioners to do so, they are accepting a type of vulnerability, thus manifesting trust. Baier refers to this as the "relative power of the truster and the trusted," and she cites the essence of trust and distrust as being the attitudes of each to the relative power and powerlessness of the trusting relation.[11]

For Baier, the cardinal features of trust include vulnerability, risk, care, and power. Reasonable trust, as opposed to blind trust or gullibility, requires having reasons for confidently expecting that others will act well. Trusting alters power positions; the position one is in without a given form of trust and the position one has within a relation of trust must be considered before one can judge whether that form of trust is essentially a relational activity. Trust often flourishes in a climate of familiarity and one's awareness of what customarily affects one's ability to trust. This has important implications for nurse-patient relationships, which often occur within larger webs of interaction. As new models of health care delivery alter the expectations of patients and other members of the health care team, there is often a lack of familiarity, and interactions are increasingly episodic rather than enduring. How is trust offered in these relationships? For some patients, it seems that trust operates as a type of faith—a leap into uncertainty, a belief on the part of the individual that the one who is trusted will act justly, thus being worthy of trust. When a trust relationship is morally sound and one can justify, on rational grounds, that the motives of the truster and trusted do not conflict harmfully, both parties are thought to have prima facie duties to preserve and protect the relationship, provided that both care about the social good that is the trust itself. This claim, of course, leads to the question of when a trusting relationship is morally sound or morally decent. For Baier, the moral test of such trust relationships is that each party be capable of surviving awareness of what the other relies on:

> ...trust is morally decent only if, in addition to whatever else is entrusted, knowledge of each party's reasons for confident reliance on the other to continue the relationship could in principle also be entrusted—since such mutual knowledge would be itself a good, not a threat to other goods. To the extent the mutual reliance can be accompanied by mutual knowledge of the conditions for that reliance, trust is above suspicion, and trustworthiness a non-suspect virtue.[11]

Applying this reasoning to the therapeutic setting, the effective therapeutic relationship should be morally good to the extent that each party relies on the other's caring, on the concern for some common good (the patient's improvement), or on the professional pride in the competent discharge of responsibility. Is this a plausible view? Does a surviving awareness of just what it is that the other is relying on in the relationship form the test of whether one can justify continued trusting and trustworthiness? It seems that something more is required. Trust is something that emerges within relationships, and implies a type of commitment toward another. One reason for justifying trust in someone is acceptance of a belief that the trusted person will choose to act for the sake of the one who risks it. Simply relying on the role-related competencies evoked by others is not the same thing as bestowing trust in them. Even assuming that caregivers are motivated by good will, something more is required for trust in them to occur. Because there is no way that cautious assessments of the trustworthiness of others can be guaranteed, trust is a risky venture, and each person wonders if bestowing trust or entrusting something of value to another is worth the associated risk. Nurse scholar Patricia Benner[12] has argued that the helping relationship requires the nurse to develop specific role-related competencies in creating a healing environment for patients and in being there for the patient as an agent of healing. These are laudable goals for holistic nursing practice, but the assumption that nurses are always worthy of the trust that such competencies would require is controversial. Because individuals have developed different trust thresholds from previous life experiences, the activity of risking trust is highly idiosyncratic, and for some individuals, trust is not welcomed.

It is clear that vulnerability is a part of the act of trusting, as is the notion that trust can be betrayed. Yet, trusting seems also to involve an optimistic belief in others, in their postulated good will, and in the epistemic confidence that trust will matter morally to others, that it will generate actions that honor vulnerability rather than abusing it or taking it for granted. To trust caregivers is to have confidence that what is entrusted to them, whether that be life, limb, or personal values and beliefs, will be respected, protected, and dignified.[13] This attitude toward entrusting is part of a network of trusting and distrusting activities that may constrain readiness to trust. Trusting, then, is an attitude toward some expected vulnerability, and it seems also to involve certain moral sanctions against the betrayal of that trust: there is a moral concern that vulnerability will be handled fairly and with respect. These sanctions, whatever they may turn out to be, are distinctly different from those legal or social sanctions, which may legitimately arise when expectations of the professed competency of another are not met. In a relationship involving trust, as opposed to one involving reliance, failure to live up to a commitment is a moral harm on the part of the trusted person, not simply a failure of role performance. Trust demands more than good will; it requires others to use their judgment and discretionary powers for moral reasons that are not simply self-serving.[14]

In summary, Baier's account of the conditions of trust and her test for the moral decency of trust are promising guidelines for showing when to bestow trust and when to withhold it. In applying her account to helping relationships in health care, important insights are offered, but it does not seem to go far enough in providing a clear distinction between trust and reliance or in establishing a clear answer to the question of what patients should expect from people that they are asked to trust. Some of the missing elements are found in the next account.

## A SOCIOLOGICAL APPROACH

Niklas Luhmann,[15] a German sociologist and attorney, published a descriptive account of trust and of power in 1973. His neofunctionalist approach to the analysis of trust and power is a highly technical yet promising endeavor. According to Luhmann, trust—in the broadest sense of confidence in one's expectations—is a basic fact of social life. He distinguishes between trust in persons and confidence in the proper operation of a system or institution. Trust is a self-evident, everyday, matter-of-fact aspect of human nature. He regards trust as vital in personal relations and a basic necessity for the derivation of rules for proper conduct:

> *If chaos and paralyzing fear are the only alternatives to trust, it follows that man, by nature, has to bestow trust, even though this is not done blindly and only in certain directions. By this method, one arrives at ethical maxims or natural law-principles, which are inherently reversible and of questionable value.*

This is so because trust emerges out of the recognition that others are free agents, free to act with their own agency. Trust occurs within a framework of interaction that is influenced by personality and social systems, and it cannot be the exclusive province of either. For Luhmann, trust goes beyond the information one has received from the past and is instead a future-oriented activity. Trust, particularly interpersonal trust, is a risky investment because it involves complex future contingencies and thus uncertainty. Although the possibilities that are part of the future are so complex, individuals seek to reduce this complexity of available choices through the act of trust. Unlike Baier, who blurs the distinction between trust and the "mere familiarity" that it presupposes, Luhmann claims that although familiarity is a necessary precondition for trust (or for distrust), it does not, in itself, provide for the occurrence of trust. This is because trust in persons is based on a deficit of complete information, and it always involves an extrapolation from whatever information is available about the person that one intends to trust. In other words, "the truster generally seeks in his subjective image of the world some objective clue about whether or not trust is justified."[15] People trust, in part, from a desire to simplify things and build relationships that are mutually supportive, rather than spending time in a state of chronic suspicion about the motives of others. Trust, then, becomes a solution to the problem of risk; it is the means to negotiate the risk associated with what is unknown about the agency and motives of others.

A vital question in this inquiry is when it is reasonable to trust others. According to Luhmann, it is not possible to demand the trust of others. Trust can only be offered and accepted. One can demand that others keep their role-related commitments and fulfill their duties, but the possibility always exists that people may choose to go outside their role boundaries. Furthermore, claims to trust cannot themselves be mechanisms for initiating or maintaining trust in others. In his view, trust is an internal mechanism and is mediated from within by the self-developing identity of the person. Trust is an attitude characterized by a blending of knowledge and ignorance; it is not transferable to others but must be an attitude which each individual develops through personal experience. The kind of trust that interests Luhmann occurs when the trusting expectation makes a difference to a decision or gives it some special significance. It overcomes an element of uncertainty in the behavior of others, about which there may always be unpredictability. Interpersonal trust is thus:

> *...the generalized expectation that the other will handle his freedom, his disturbing potential for diverse actions, in keeping with his personality—or rather, in keeping with the personality which he has presented and made socially visible. He who stands by what he has allowed to be known about himself, whether consciously or unconsciously, is worthy of trust.*[15]

Luhmann identifies 3 stages for initiating trust between persons. In the first, there has to be some cause for displaying trust, some situation in which the truster depends on the trustee. This psychological requirement involves a commitment to risk and a recognition that one's vulnerability is the instrument by which a trust relationship can be created. Thus, individuals learn how to trust, and they learn that it is possible for that trust to be abused. The second stage involves a cognitive assessment based on easily interpretable situations, involving the possibility of communication and including the precondition of familiarity. This stage involves a shift from the external to the internal, whereby the readiness to trust is equated with the degree of self-confidence possessed by the person. For Luhmann, this includes an assessment of those "socially visible" attributes that a person presents, either as a personality character- istic or as a set of normative role expectations. In the third stage, Luhmann discusses the process by which trust can become the object of norms. It involves a reference back to the external social environment for the purpose of gaining symbolic control over the object of trust. If expectations regarding the prospects for gain or loss and the unequal distributions of power are stabilized, then the conditions for mutuality of trustworthy commitment are established.

The ingredients of the trust formation process, as depicted by Luhmann, have important implications for the helping relationship in nursing and other professions. Luhmann sees a delicacy in human relations, where tact is used in presenting oneself to another so that offers of trust-engaging behavior can be accepted or rejected without fear of hostility. In his view, the basis for all trust is the presentation of the indi- vidual self as a social identity, and trust builds itself up through interactions with others and with the social environment. Trust in one's own self-presentation or role perfor- mance, and in others' interpretations of it, gives rise to occasions for increasing trust. Similarly, in his view, the inability to show trust, by failing to present oneself confidently to another, reduces the chances for winning or earning trust. When trust between people is not possible or justified, they end up simply cooperating with each other under some negotiated system of rules or regulations. In summary, Luhmann offers an important analysis of the phenomenon of trust in persons and the related notion of confidence in institutions or systems. Clearly, the connection drawn between risk and trust has implications for understanding the helping role in nurse-patient interac- tions. It illustrates that an individual can initially place trust in a system or institution and its representatives rather than in a particular individual. This has important impli- cations for health care institutions and professions, in that it demonstrates the instru- mental value of social trust in public life and organizational ethics. The generalized confidence in the functional capacities of nursing as a helping profession or in the effi- cient operation of a familiar structure, such as a hospital, is not trust in the strict sense, but it may influence the point at which trust is offered, tempered, withheld, or with- drawn. Patients may thus have a general readiness to trust nurses as members of a trusted profession, insofar as they rely on the social attributes and role performance of its members. However, this is not interpersonal trust.

The placement of trust in an individual nurse is a different matter—one that relates to the question of whether a specific nurse will act in the patient's best interests when those interests have not been clearly specified in advance. Nurse scholar de Raeve[16] argues that trust is fostered not merely by reliance on the professional competencies of nurses but rather by the attitude of "caring about" patients instead of simply "caring for" them. Caring about patients, she says, "seems to require some reflective scrutiny of motives and reactions on the part of the nurse and some active moral commitment to try to see patients with attitudes of generosity, charity, and compassion." She recognizes that the trust that patients place in nurses is often without knowledge of their specific trustworthiness as individuals; patients often have to trust nurses even when a relationship has yet to form. Without caring about patients and helping them, nurses may always be in danger of breaching the trust invested in them.[16] It is clear that trust is vital to interpersonal relationships in nursing. And yet, trust between people is not always possible; it can be elusive, unwarranted, and even abused. Studies indicate that organizations desirous of earning the highest levels of trust, based on shared values with those whom they serve, will need to go beyond minimum standards of truthfulness and confidence in their functional capacities or role performance indicators.[17] Trust and trustworthiness, whether in individuals or institutions, require an acceptance and negotiation of the asymmetry of power, knowledge, and agency, which are inherent in different forms of trust behavior.

## THE PARENT-CHILD MODEL OF TRUST

This model is familiar to most psychologists and social theorists as presented in the "Eight Ages of Man" chapter of Erikson's *Childhood and Society*, first published in 1950.[18] Erikson elucidates the psycho-social-sexual developmental tasks that individuals exhibit as they mature into adulthood. Maturation for Erikson is essentially a search for ego integrity. Each stage is marked by a task that is either affirmed or negated. The stage concerned with trust formation is the first and most general stage, called "Basic Trust vs. Basic Mistrust". As will be seen, trust in this model is limited to an individual psychological orientation that is tied to the early socialization experiences of the individual. Erikson postulates a general encounter between the child's maturing ego and the social world. In the initial phase, as infants try to take in the things they need, they interact with caretakers. These caretakers are part of a socio-cultural milieu and exhibit certain developed preferences and values in their behavior of giving and caring. Most important in these interactions is that infants come to find some consistency, predictability, and reliability in their caretakers' nurturing and benevolent actions. When they sense that a parent is consistent and dependable and that provisions will be made to relieve the discomfort of cold, hunger, and threat, infants develop a sense of trust. Although some parents respond on demand and others on some prescribed schedule, infants learn that the parent is dependable and therefore worthy of basic trust. Any negotiation of these expectations fosters mistrust, and thus the infant learns about uncertainty and vulnerability. This process allows the individual to differentiate situations of both trust and mistrust, and Erikson claims "it is clear that the human infant must experience a goodly measure of mistrust to trust discerningly."[18] For Erikson, it is clear that encounters between parent and child are not necessarily blissful ones; rather, these encounters lead to acquired expectations of certain behaviors, such as comfort, satisfaction, security, or their opposites.

Although trust, for Erikson, depends on a sense of reliability and prediction, he feels that something more is required. He says that trust ultimately depends on the parents' own confidence, on their sense that they are doing things right. Parents "must be able to represent to the child a deep, almost somatic conviction that there is a meaning to what they are doing."[18] This sense of meaning, in turn, requires cultural backing—the belief that "the way we do things is good for our children."[18] Parents and caretakers can gain confidence from their faith in some aspects of their culture, which may include the simple advice to go ahead and follow their inclinations to meet the infant's biological and psychological needs. In this social aspect, Erikson broadens Freud's description of the libidinal zone considerably, and he sees the infant's oral behaviors of sucking, biting, and grasping as ways of integrating the developing sense of self with the world. One cannot read Erikson without appreciating the elegance of his theory (presented here only in part) and his descriptions of the utterly dependent infant embarking on the first stages of social interaction. Many health care providers and patients have adopted, if somewhat instinctively, this parent-child model. Some do so because they prefer more paternalistic models of patient interaction, in that such models often ensure unquestioning compliance, unilateral trust, and a regressive dependency.

## MODELS OF TRUST IN MEDICINE

Many of the ideas emerging from these models are exemplified in the work of Talcott Parsons,[19] best known for his discussion on the concept of the "sick role" in medicine. Although inadequate in many respects, Parson's sociological perspective does represent a still prevalent attitude regarding the nature of patient-physician relationships and the elements of trust said to be inherent in them. He advocates a formal and distant stance between the physician and patient, yet one in which both are collectively united in the goal of therapy. In the following statement we note the quick shift from mutual trust to authority that has often appeared in these justifications:

> [T]he patient is expected to "have confidence" in his physician, and if this confidence breaks down, to seek another physician. This may be interpreted to mean that the relationship is expected to be one of mutual "trust," of the belief that the physician is trying his best to help the patient and that, conversely, the patient is "cooperating" with him to the best of his ability. [T]he doctor-patient relationship has to be one involving an element of authority.[19]

Parson's view expresses an attitude still shared by many physicians. Trust, on this account, is the "something" that bridges the gap of competence between the superordinate physician and the relatively helpless patient. The patient is thus obligated to rely on the physician without ever having the opportunity, or not perhaps until recently, to evaluate these claims for expertise and esoteric knowledge.

It is often the case that such a model also appeals to patients. For instance, in *The Silent World of Doctor and Patient*, Jay Katz[20] writes:

> It appealed to patients, engulfed by pain and suffering, because surrender to powerful, wise, and soothing caretakers was strongly fostered by memories of earlier days when a parent satisfied all discomforting bodily needs. Thus, the regression to more childlike functioning that can result from illness becomes augmented by a patient's wish for caretaking by a parent-physician who, as memory informs, will immediately alleviate all suffering. The regression is also reinforced by doctors' proclivities to view patients as helpless and incompetent children.

Katz goes on to deny the utility of the parent-child model of trust for adult patients, and he argues instead for a model of shared authority between patient and practitioners. He challenges the traditional view that patients should trust their physicians because their physicians have more competent knowledge of medicine and what constitutes the patients' best interests. Although the substance of these claims is certainly questionable, the medical profession has undoubtedly purposively construed the concept of trust as an obligation the patient should have toward the physician.[21-23] His alternative model, developed primarily for physicians but also useful to nursing professionals, is based on "the confident and trusting expectation that physicians will assist patients to make their own decisions—decisions that, in the light of their medical needs and personal history, they deem to be in their best interests".[20] Trust cannot be earned through deeds alone but must be verbally communicated in a purposeful dialog, according to Katz. There should be a willingness on the part of practitioners to share the burden of decision-making with patients and to acknowledge their own limits—whether in scientific knowledge or in their own personal incapacities. In this egalitarian view, physicians earn the trust of patients by placing trust in the patients themselves. Although this approach may have important philosophical merit, its clinical applicability may be restricted to various contextual concerns. Nevertheless, it illustrates an important element of the role of personal belief in matters related to the process of trust. When ill, people do depend on the technical knowledge and professional skills of their providers, to regain health, function, hope, or a sense of value. Often they are placed in situations where they are expected to have a "confident reliance on the other." This confidence has been encouraged by health professions through promotion of an ideology of altruistic service to others and through claims regarding the possession of a great body of esoteric knowledge that supposedly is unattainable to the public.

## TRUST MATTERS IN NURSING

The preceding discussion demonstrates that trust is an attitude held toward those who are expected to be trustworthy. Trust is a complex process of internal mediation, which incorporates risk and vulnerability whenever a future action or decision that one cares about is encountered. This mediation might well result in decisions to withhold one's trust or even to mistrust another for prudent reasons. Some have argued that we should place trust in others with care and discernment, acknowledging that there is never a guarantee that breaches of trust will not occur.[11,24] Others remind us that trust may be a solution to the problem of risk and uncertainty, but trust never eliminates all risk of disappointment. Trust in the nursing profession is based on the assumption that its members are able and willing to use their power to advance the good that it aims to bring about. What makes this assumption valid? How do issues of professional power and authority affect the morality of the trust relationship?

At the core of helping relationships in health care is asymmetry or inequality between the helper and the help seeker and in the latter's dependence on the former. This asymmetry creates special demands on the integrity of the helper and the professional attitude the helper uses in terms of power. The most important characteristic in this imbalance between helpers and help seekers is the element of trust, and it can sometimes be a feeding ground for inappropriate motivations and strategies. In *The Magnetism of Power in Helping Relationships and Asymmetry*, Schuyt[25] notes that the "helping professions" such as nursing can attract people who "may be lured, knowingly or unknowingly, by the position of authority, by the dependence of others, by the image of benevolence, by the promise of adulation, or by a hope of vicariously helping themselves through helping others." In dealing with these inequalities and possible abuses of power, it is essential that nurses develop skills to set appropriate boundaries for their interactions with patients, and to act in ways that honor the patient's need.

Although illness expresses itself in diverse ways, most ill people demonstrate the following characteristics: feelings of dependence; the need for control, comfort, protection, and help; and a desire to have these needs met in a culturally respectful manner. Patients become dependent on others in ways that may threaten their sense of autonomy and independence. This can lead to feelings of vulnerability, which further deepens issues such as the readiness to trust others. Patients are most vulnerable when illness and other conditions do not allow them to be autonomous or self-regulative. In other words, when individuals can no longer direct the path of their own life or determine the goals that give life meaning, they become more vulnerable. This lack of control sometimes means that patients have no option except to rely on others, especially when illness or injury has eroded their sense of safety, self-efficacy, or sense of future. This often exacerbates the vulnerability and risks brought on by the illness experience, especially when the initial encounter between a nurse and patient is that of strangers. According to ethicist Howard Brody[26], shared power reduces the distance between professional and patient and allows for the possibility of understanding the encounter between them as an opportunity for growth and development for both. He acknowledges that the degree to which the professional understands the power differential inherent in the helping role, and the communication associated with sharing this power with patients, influences the ethical dimensions of the encounter between them. Thus, given the inherent asymmetry in professional-patient relationships in general, the unequal distribution of power, and the feelings of vulnerability often invoked in the patient by the illness experience, it is clear that building a trusting relationship with patients is a moral and healing art.

## SUMMARY

Responsible helping is not simply the possession of knowledge or expertise; it emerges from the identity and integrity of the helper. Indeed, as Nightingale[27] says, the nurse is the caregiver who is principally responsible for creating a healing environment. This assumes a sense of moral agency on the part of the nurse that extends beyond the notion of role performance or technical skill. Helping is not only what the nurse accomplishes in meeting the needs of the patient but also incorporates a way of being. Trust is a relational process, one that is dynamic and fragile, yet involving the deepest needs and vulnerabilities of individuals. These needs and vulnerabilities are remarkably reflexive, often changing with age, illness, and successful (or unsuccessful) encounters with others. Trust enables nurses and other health care professionals to respond morally to the needs of patients and is thus a vital dimension of clinical practice. By navigating the moral landscape of trust, vulnerability, power, and helping, the concept of trust acquires a normative position in nursing. In its moral dimension, trust invokes an element of intrinsic value, not merely a factual exchange between persons or an instrumental good. It is even more fundamental than duties of beneficence, veracity, and nonmaleficence, because without trust, nobody would have a reason to take on these duties in the first place (Carter MA. [1989]. Ethical analysis of trust in therapeutic relationships; unpublished doctoral dissertation, University of Tennessee, Knoxville).

## REFERENCES

1. Wiedenbach E. Clinical nursing, a helping art. New York: Springer Publishing Co; 1964.
2. Koloroutis M, Manthey M, Felgen J, et al. Relationship-based care, a model for transforming practice. Minneapolis (MN): Creative Health Care Management; 2004.
3. Medias EP. Reciprocity in the healing relationship between nurse and patient. In: Kritek P, editor. Reflections on healing: a central nursing construct. New York: NLN press; 1997. p. 435–51.
4. Hood L, Leddy S. Professional communication to establish helping and healing relationships. In: Hood LJ, Leddy SK, editors. Leddy and Pepper's conceptual bases of professional nursing. 6th edition. Philadelphia: Lippincott, Williams & Wilkins; 2006. p. 168–200.
5. Tschirch P. Nightingale on healing. In: Kritek PB, editor. Reflections on healing: a central nursing construct. New York: NLN Press; 1997. p. 43–55.

6. Hupcey JE, Penrod J, Morse JM, et al. An exploration and advancement of the concept of trust. J Adv Nurs 2001;36:282–93.

7. Shore DA. The trust crisis in healthcare, causes, consequences, and cures. New York: Oxford University Press; 1997.

8. Bok S. Lying: moral choice in public and private life. New York: Pantheon Books; 1978.

9. Gallop Honesty/Ethics in Professions Poll. (n.d.). Available at: http://www.gallup.com/poll/1654/Honesty-ethics-professions.aspx. Accessed November 7, 2008.

10. Baier A. Postures of the mind: essays on mind and morals. Minneapolis (MN): University of Minnesota Press; 1985.

11. Baier A. Trust and anti-trust. Ethics 1986;96:231–60.

12. Benner P. From novice to expert: excellence and power in clinical nursing practice. Menlo Park (CA): Addison-Wesley; 1984.

13. Carter MA. Ethical framework for care of the chronically ill. Holistic Nursing Practice 1993;8:67–77.

14. McLeod C. Self-trust and reproductive autonomy. Cambridge: The MIT Press; 2002.

15. Luhmann N. Trust and power. New York: John Wiley and Sons; 1979.

16. de Raeve L. Trust and trustworthiness in nurse-patient relationships. Nursing Philosophy 2002;3:152–62.

17. Gould S, Klipp G. Managed care members talk about trust. Soc Sci Med 2002;54: 879–88.

18. Erikson EH. Childhood and society. 2nd edition. New York: W.W. Norton and Co; 1963.

19. Parsons T. The social system. New York: The Free Press; 1951.

20. Katz J. The silent world of doctor and patient. New York: The Free Press; 1984.

21. Starr P. The social transformation of American medicine. New York: Basic Books; 1982.

22. Mechanic D. Physicians and patients in transition. Hastings Cent Rep 1985;15: 9–12.

23. Freidson E. Professional dominance: the social structure of medical care. New York: Atherton; 1970.

24. O'Neill O. Autonomy and trust in bioethics. Cambridge: Cambridge University Press; 2002.

25. Schuyt T. The magnetism of power in helping relationships. Professional attitude and asymmetry. Social Work and Society 2004;2:39–53. Available at: www.socwork.de/Schuyt2004.pdf.

26. Brody H. Yale University Press; 1992.

27. Nightingale F. Notes on nursing: what it is, and what it is not. New York: Appleton & Company; 1860.

# Personal Conscience and the Problem of Moral Certitude

Cheryl Ellis Vaiani, PhD

KEYWORDS

• Moral certainty • Personal integrity
• Professional integrity • Moral agency

## MORAL CERTAINTY

*It's not what we don't know that gets us in trouble, it's what we know for SURE that just ain't true…*

*Mark Twain*

Moral certainty, very simply, is knowing that you are right. The answer is a "sure thing," a foregone conclusion. Moral certainty is founded on an absolute belief to which the person is committed, without doubt.[1–3] For some, religion provides moral certainty. Those who believe in religion trust that the written or spoken word and teachings of a supreme being are absolutely correct. An adherent to those teachings acts in good conscience according to those beliefs.

A look back through history is replete with examples of wars fought and injustices applied to impose or compel specific beliefs. Whether religious or ideologic, the certainty that only one's beliefs are correct and must at all costs be forced on others is alarming. Seeing the world as simply black or white, right or wrong may provide individuals reassuring certainty about their actions, but it also negates the need for critical, reflective thinking that enhances ethical practice.

The moral practice of nursing requires the difficult work of discerning the best response to an ethical quandary. Determining the right course of action can rarely be discovered by assuming that one value, one theory, one point of view will always and reliably identify the morality of an action. Although moral ambiguity brings with it the need to question, investigate, and delve deeper into moral dilemmas, it is an essential aspect of moral behavior. Ethical theories and methods, such as principalism, Kantian ethics, casuistry, utilitarianism, narrative ethics, virtue ethics, feminist ethics, and phenomenology, may shed moral knowledge on the question. The right course of action should reflect previous cases, laws, and decisions, but there are

Institute for the Medical Humanities, University of Texas Medical Branch, 301 University Boulevard, Route 1311, Galveston, TX 77555-1311, USA
*E-mail address:* cevaiani@utmb.edu

Nurs Clin N Am 44 (2009) 407–414
doi:10.1016/j.cnur.2009.07.008
0029-6465/09/$ – see front matter © 2009 Elsevier Inc. All rights reserved.

always particulars to the situation that must be discovered, examined, and considered. Moral perception, reflection, and action concerning complex dilemmas of practice are all demanding work. Practitioners who move too quickly to a state of moral certainty about a decision may be missing essential components of the enactment of moral agency.

Mary Ellen Wurzbach, a professor of nursing at the University of Wisconsin Oshkosh, has examined the moral behavior of nurses regarding the concept of moral certainty. Her research has documented that moral certainty is a common experience for nurses and serves to provide comfort and prompt action. Wurzbach[4–6] described morally certain nurses as "knowing the thing to do" without needing to check with a colleague or to question their beliefs. But a nurse's moral certainty brings with it a risk of stifling dialog and in-depth discussion of moral issues. How can one tell the difference between unjustified action based upon unproven enthusiasm or self-deception and justified action based on reflective moral conviction?

Philosopher Lichtenburg suggests the development of an attitude of detachment from one's own beliefs so that one might see the possibility of being "blinded by passions, interests, upbringing and might be mistaken."[7] Because moral certainty does not guarantee a positive or appropriate outcome, seeking moral resolution requires questioning, investigating, and considering possible alternative views or actions. To achieve such a reflective moral stance, Wurzbach suggests the necessary virtues and actions for nurses:

> Although the virtues of persistence, patience, and commitment lead toward moral clarity, I caution nurses not to be satisfied with certainty. Appreciate, cultivate, and welcome the moral uncertainty and ambiguity that you experience along the way. Take the path toward moral clarity, but appreciate the journey.[8]

## CONFRONTING ETHICAL DILEMMAS

A physician author, writing about stress and distress in nurses, agrees that health care professionals are confronted daily with ethical dilemmas as part of their clinical practice. He attests that it is important that they scrutinize their judgments, attitudes, and actions. This critical, reflective thinking enhances ethical practice and ensures that decisions are based on professional, ethical, and moral principles rather than on personal biases or preferences.[9] Unless nurses are aware of the personal emotions, values, and priorities that they bring to the clinical encounter, they may "exchange ethical deliberation for moral dogma,"[10] and therefore fail to consider other important goals and values. Most human beings and particularly those in the helping professions want to think that they are good people doing the right thing, and it is tempting to have "the right answer."

Moral judgment involves integrating numerous ethical considerations that count for or against a particular course or action to decide what should be done in a specific situation. The moral tension involved in this reflective exercise is often characterized by feelings of anxiety, intellectual perplexity, conflict, emotional vulnerability, ambivalence, being overwhelmed, and a lack of clarity. On the other hand, certitude reduces or eliminates ambiguity, allows one to know where she or he stands, is efficient, does not require consideration of particulars or context, makes one feel good about oneself, and protects and confirms one's image as a good person. Although in this comparison certitude might seem a better state, Churchill submits that moral tension is inherent in the human condition. There is always a pull between who we are and who we hope to be, and because of the temporal quality of moral judgments, our knowledge is partial and opaque. To Churchill, moral judgments are not guarantees of moral correctness, and therefore they require ethical reflection.[11]

## CASE STUDY

Several years ago, I was contacted by the director of nursing of a community hospital with a report of an incident that had occurred in the obstetrics unit. She reported that a patient, approximately 14 to 16 weeks pregnant, had presented to the hospital with grossly ruptured membranes. The obstetrician caring for the patient believed that the patient would most certainly lose the pregnancy, called it an inevitable abortion, and recommended that steps be taken to terminate the pregnancy to protect the mother from infection and preserve her future reproductive potential. The patient agreed to her physician's recommendations. When the physician ordered the necessary steps to begin, the nurses on duty refused to be involved in any way with the termination of the pregnancy. The nurses stated that they would gladly "care" for the patient but insisted that they would only participate in efforts to preserve the pregnancy. Unable to find any nurses who would participate in the plan of care, the patient was transferred to another hospital. The director of nursing was worried and concerned about the actions of the nurses and requested that I meet with the obstetric nursing staff to discuss the issues.

About a week later, I met with approximately 15 nurses assigned to the obstetrics area. My plan was to engage the nurses in a conversation about nursing responsibility, patient autonomy, and conflicts that might exist between personal beliefs and professional actions. My hope was to encourage reflection, dialog, and discussion of possible alternatives to their chosen action, to consider ambiguity and nuance in their moral thinking, and to cultivate questioning and investigation as aspects of moral behavior.

I fear that I failed miserably in my goals. I was met with an attitude that I can only describe as one of moral certainty. The nurses, at least the ones who spoke up, were clearly proud of their actions and absolutely certain that they were correct. Although some mentioned a religious source for their certainty, others held up one of their own, as an example of good, even expected character. "X has struggled with a child with special needs, worked full time, and is a single mother. This mother should be willing to do the same." What these nurses seemed steadfastly unwilling to consider was that any other perspective was worth their consideration.

### Discussion

This case study presents multiple issues. Personal integrity and professional integrity, patient interests, society's expectation of a profession, the balance between rights and obligations within the nurse-patient relationship, acting according to one's conscience, power, control, and moral certainty are but a few of the topics to consider. Examination of these topics sheds light on the current debate about professional conscience clauses but more than that encourages reflection and dialog by the practitioners of nursing. These topics promise to enrich thinking about the moral richness of nursing practice and will encourage readers to know, to reason, and to act in ways that demonstrate reflective moral judgment.

In their attitude of moral certainty, perhaps, the nurses in the case mentioned earlier did not give enough consideration to patient autonomy, dignity, or well-being. Perhaps they lost sight of their professional role in enabling or helping the patient achieve her goals, or maybe they saw their personal beliefs or conscience as more important or convincing. It is the tension between personal and professional integrity and conscience that may offer further insight into this case.

## THE CLINICAL SITUATION

Before moving to the distinctly moral issues, the clinical details of the situation of the case must be briefly presented. To make the best ethical decisions concerning health care, it is essential that the clinical facts be correct. How realistic were the chances of continuing this pregnancy to deliver a viable infant? What were the health risks to the mother, and how serious were they?

Premature rupture of membranes is defined as rupture of the membranes before the start of labor in a close-to-term pregnancy (>37 weeks) and is considered to be a normal physiologic process. Preterm premature rupture of membranes (PPROM) or rupture of membranes before 37 weeks can result from a wide array of pathologic mechanisms and is typically associated with a brief latency period between membrane rupture and delivery, increased potential for perinatal infection, and in utero cord compression. Management hinges on careful evaluation of the gestational age and balancing the relative risks of preterm birth versus intrauterine infection, abruptio placentae, and cord accident with expectant management. The risk of intra-amniotic infection is 13% to 60% and that of postpartum infection is 2.8% to 13%, with increasing incidence of infection with decreasing gestational age at rupture.[12]

Management of rupture of membranes before fetal viability is particularly controversial and complicated. Viability is a dynamic concept and is affected by several factors; most consider pregnancies less than 24 completed weeks to be previable because anatomic development of the lungs cannot support air exchange.[13] Some sources suggest that incomplete abortion is a more appropriate term for those pregnancies when PPROM has occurred before 20 weeks, because the products of conception (amniotic fluid) have passed the cervical opening and into the vagina.[14] Regardless, these immature pregnancies are considered to have a poor, even dismal, prognosis, and although pregnancy prolongation and neonatal survival is possible, the morbidity remains high.[15] When PPROM occurs before 20 weeks' gestation, the probability of reaching viability is less than 5%,[16] and some data indicate 20 weeks to be a turning point in neonatal survival.[17] Although the complications of prematurity are extensive and well known, pregnancies with PPROM before 24 weeks have the additional risk of lethal pulmonary hypoplasia secondary to prolonged, severe, early oligohydramnios.[18]

In gestations less than 24 weeks with PPROM, the American College of Obstetricians and Gynecologists suggests that either expectant management or induction of labor are treatment options, and patients should be counseled on their potential risks and benefits. Expectant management would most likely include bed rest, complete pelvic rest, periodic monitoring, and perhaps long-term hospitalization. Typically, after an initial period of hospitalization after rupture of membranes, patients with previable pregnancies are followed as outpatients and readmitted to hospital once the pregnancy has reached the limit of viability. Because the best chance of fetal survival depends on the immediate availability of obstetric monitoring and neonatal intensive care facilities, the patient should ideally be managed in close proximity to those services. It is important that patients considering expectant management be well informed and educated about their personal risks, the costs, and the commitment required in attempting to continue the pregnancy and also about the extremely poor prognosis for the neonate.[19] These are formidable decisions for patients and clinicians. For the subgroup with gestations less than 20 weeks potential maternal complications may outweigh the minimal chance of neonatal survival. Long-term maternal hospitalization, infection risk, high rate of cesarean delivery, and neonatal morbidity[20] can be significant burdens to the patient and would seem to indicate that the decision should remain with those who will bear the burdens.

## CONSCIENCE AND CONSCIENTIOUS OBJECTION

Although recent controversies regarding pharmacists refusing to prescribe or dispense contraceptives have sparked a renewed debate about conscientious objection in health care, conscience clauses have been common since *Roe v Wade*. Abortion, blood transfusion, withholding and withdrawing life support (particularly artificially provided nutrition and hydration), organ donation, assisted suicide, contraception and/or family planning interventions, and even unsafe staffing conditions are areas in which nurses can be confronted with difficult decisions. Rather than trying to address the larger debate, the focus here is on examination of the conflict between professional role and personal conscience in nurses in the case discussed earlier.

Nursing history and foundational documents provide the nurse with resources that can be used for ethical inquiry. At least from the time of Florence Nightingale, nursing has emphasized wholeness or holistic practice that includes a responsibility of self-care for the nurse as an essential component. Nightingale believed that integrity, being personally responsible for personal moral conduct, was part of a nurse's wholeness.[21,22] The American Nurses Association (ANA) code of ethics, scope and standards of practice, and social policy statement facilitate ethical decision making for practicing nurses. The code of ethics documents and establishes the core moral values of the profession and outlines the important values, duties, and responsibilities that are inherent in the role of the nurse. According to the ANA, the code is "a succinct statement of the ethical obligations and duties" of the nurse, "the profession's non-negotiable ethical standards," and "an expression of nursing's own understanding of its commitment."[23] The first 3 provisions of the code are identified as describing "the most fundamental values and commitments of the nurse."[24] Those provisions are compassion and respect for the dignity of every individual, the obligations to the patient, and being a patient advocate. The primacy of these duties would clearly be applicable to moral questions about conflicts between personal and professional promises. The code is unusual in that it also recognizes specifically a nurse's obligations to self, in sections 5.3 and 5.4. A nurse is responsible to care for personal health, rights, and moral integrity. Although the code does not explicitly state a hierarchy of these duties, obligations to the patient might be inferred as primary. Clearly the ANA code recognizes the potential conflict between personal and professional values.

Quinn and Smith, in *The Professional Commitment: Issues and Ethics in Nursing*, assert that uncertainty is inherent in professional nursing. They contend that nurses must address uncertainty through open communication with fellow nurses, by developing skills in moral reasoning, and by applying ethical principles to clinical situations.[25] Benjamin and Curtis outline 3 conditions for appeals to conscience in nursing. In order for a refusal to count, it must be (1) personal and subjective, based on standards one does not necessarily apply to others, (2) founded on a prior judgment of rightness or wrongness, and (3) motivated by personal sanction rather than external authority.[26]

Although individuals clearly should be guided by their convictions, that does not necessarily make their convictions correct or their behavior morally right. Reasoning about what makes behavior morally right should have an answer other than "my conscience tells me so." Because claiming a conscientious objection, in essence, tells others that they are wrong, nurses should be expected to specify and articulate concerns, values, and principles that make an action, in their view, right or wrong.[27]

Howard Brody has written on the difference between personal and professional integrity in a way that brings clarity to the situation. He contends that as members of a profession, nurses have made a public and collective promise to place the interests of the patient above their own self-interest. Nurses therefore have role responsibilities that society expects they should fulfill because they have promised to do so. When nurses claim a conscientious objection, their personal and professional integrity are in conflict. But which type of integrity should take precedence? According to Brody, individuals have a complex set of moral commitments that they seek to balance to achieve integrity or wholeness. He suggests that, "…we can hardly ever be single-issue voters. Therefore, an apparently conscientious judgment may turn out to be flawed as a result of not truly representing our whole set of important moral commitments."[28]

## REFLECTIVE ANALYSIS

When the nurses acted out their personal conscience by refusing to participate in what they interpreted as an act of abortion, they subjected the patient to negative actions that may not have been consistent with even their own moral commitments or conscience. Their actions coerced the patient into a plan she and her doctor did not choose, increased the patient's level of stress, made the patient's transfer necessary (thereby increasing emotional and financial costs), compromised patient dignity, and placed her well-being at risk by subjecting her to the physical risks (infection, sepsis, even death) of a treatment plan she did not choose. By demanding that the patient attempt to preserve the pregnancy, the nurses ignored many other basic moral commitments and promises they swore to uphold, such as patient autonomy, dignity, and well-being. Although they did not directly abandon their patient, they certainly used their professional power to control and limit her choices. Imagining a single moral dictate as a sole commitment fails to consider or give weight to other important goals and values that nurses might regard as part of their personal or professional integrity. When examined in this way, individual conscience may not provide clarity or certainty to moral decision making; instead it serves as a "trump card" that may lead to questionable decisions. The dictates of conscience are morally weighty, but so are professional responsibilities.

When nurses give their conscience authority over their professional nursing role, they neglect a fundamental, central value of nursing. Card[29] has suggested that the moral center of professionalism is the primacy of patient interests. Imposing personal views on a patient who is dependent and vulnerable would seem to betray that value and commitment. The right to conscience is abused when it compels others to comply involuntarily with a belief that they do not share. After all, the assumption should be that the patient is acting according to her conscience also.

Nurses must learn to balance their rights and obligations within the nurse-patient relationship and accomplish the difficult work of moral inquiry. The individual nurse must decide how to rank her many competing values and beliefs to determine which best satisfies all of her core moral responsibilities. The hope is that the individual nurse would be able to resolve this moral quandary without being put in the position of having to decide whether to be an ethical nurse or an ethical person, there may well be certain consciences that are not suited for certain roles. For example, a nurse who is an adherent of the Jehovah's Witness faith and feels herself unable to participate, perhaps even touch blood for transfusion, may not be suited for employment in an emergency department or intensive care unit where that duty is frequently required.

In cases where the conscientious objection may have less effect on her role, the individual nurse not only has the responsibility to declare her objection upon employment but also to participate in a plan with the management to limit its effect on patient care. Although institutional or systems-level policies attempt to resolve such issues by replacing the objecting practitioner with someone willing to perform the service, such resolution works best with the flexibility provided by large institutions. In smaller hospitals, isolated areas, or in situations where trained staff seem to have decided as a group not to provide a particular service, the resolution is more challenging. In these more unusual cases, nurses' right to conscientious objection must be invoked in a way that allows patients to have access to nursing care and achieve their goals.

## SUMMARY

The role of the nurse is an inherently moral activity that is at the heart and soul of health care. Patients understand the role of the nurse as being to protect, advocate, and assist the patient in achieving their goals, and they would be perplexed, even deceived, by a nurse or group of nurses who obstructed the agreed plan of care. Provision 2 of the *Code of Ethics for Nurses* leaves little doubt: "The nurses' primary commitment is to the recipient of nursing and health care services – the patient – whether the recipient is an individual, family, group, or a community … the nurse strives to provide patients with the opportunity to participate in planning care, assures that patients find the plan acceptable, and supports the implementation of the plan."[30]

Reflecting on the actions of the nurses in the case recounted at the beginning of this article raises serious concerns. In an attempt to maintain their personal integrity, it seems the nurses lost sight of the patient and their own professional integrity. Their moral certainty about the right course of action and seeming inability to reflect on alternate values and actions challenges the idea that they have done the work of moral inquiry or even realized that reflection was part of their moral agency. Although, perhaps not surprisingly, considering the political and religious rhetoric that surrounds abortion today, it is distressing that nurses who pride themselves on being the caring profession could seemingly refuse to reflect on their moral judgments or discuss what duty they owed to the patient.

## REFERENCES

1. Miller R. Absolute certainty. Mind 1978;87:46–65.
2. Klein P. Certainty: a refutation of skepticism. Minneapolis (MN): University of Minnesota Press; 1981.
3. Lichtenburg J. Moral certainty. Philosophy 1994;69:181–204.
4. Wurzbach M. Acute care nurses' experiences of moral certainty. J Adv Nurs 1999; 30(2):287–93.
5. Wurzbach M. Long-term care nurses' ethical convictions about tube-feeding. West J Nurs Res 1996;18(1):63–76.
6. Wurzbach M. Long-term care nurses' moral convictions. J Adv Nurs 1995;21(6): 1059–64.
7. Lichtenburg J. Moral certainty. Philosophy 1994;69:182.
8. Wurzbach M. Doing what's right: the ethics of nursing. Reflect Nurs Leadersh 2005;31(3):1–4.
9. Perkin R. Stress and distress in pediatric nurses: the hidden tragedy of baby k. Loma Linda University Bioethics Update 1996;12(2):1–9.
10. Churchill L, Siman J. Principles and the search for moral certainty. Soc Sci Med 1986;23(5):461–8.

11. Churchill L, Siman J. Principles and the search for moral certainty. Soc Sci Med 1986;23(5):465.
12. ACOG Committee on Practice Bulletins-Obstetrics. ACOG practice bulletin no. 80: premature rupture of membranes. Clinical management guidelines for obstetrician-gynecologists. Obstet Gynecol 2007;109(4):1007–19.
13. Higgins R, Papadopoulos M, Raju T. Executive summary of the workshop on the border of viability. Pediatrics 2005;115:1392–6.
14. Jazayeri A. Premature rupture of membranes in emedicine. Available at: http://emedicine.medscape.com/article/261137-overview. Accessed January 20, 2009.
15. Dinsmoor MJ, Bachman R, Haney EI, et al. Outcomes after expectant management of extremely preterm premature rupture of the membranes. Am J Obstet Gynecol 2004;190(1):183–7.
16. Mercer B, Milluzzi C, Collin M. Previable birth at 20 to 26 weeks of gestation: proximate causes, previous obstetric history and recurrence risk. Am J Obstet Gynecol 2005;193(3 Pt 2):1175–80.
17. Falk S, Campbell L, Lee-Parritz A, et al. Expectant management in spontaneous preterm premature rupture of membranes between 14 and 24 weeks' gestation. J Perinatol 2004;24(10):611–6.
18. ACOG Committee on Practice Bulletins-Obstetrics. ACOG practice bulletin no. 80: premature rupture of membranes. Clinical management guidelines for obstetrician-gynecologists. Obstet Gynecol 2007;109(4):1009.
19. ACOG Committee on Practice Bulletins-Obstetrics. ACOG practice bulletin no. 80: premature rupture of membranes. Clinical management guidelines for obstetrician-gynecologists. Obstet Gynecol 2007;109(4):1014.
20. Grisaru-Granovsky S, Eitan R, Kaplan M, et al. Expectant management of mid-trimester premature rupture of membranes: a plea for limits. J Perinatol 2003; 23:235–9.
21. Dorsey B, Selanders L, Beck, D, et al. Florence Nightingale today; healing, leadership, global action. Silver Spring (MD): American Nurses Association; 2005. p. 49, 52–3.
22. Ulrich B. Leadership and management according to Florence Nightingale. Norwalk (CT): Appleton & Lange; 1992. p. 51.
23. American Nurses Association. Code of ethics with interpretive statements. 2001. Nursing World Website. Available at: http://nursingworld.org/ethics/code/protected_nwcoe813.htm. Accessed January 30, 2009.
24. American Nurses Association. Code of ethics with interpretive statements. 2001. Nursing World Website. Available at: http://nursingworld.org/ethics/code/protected_nwcoe813.htm. Accessed January 30, 2009.
25. Quinn C, Smith M. The professional commitment: issues and ethics in nursing. Philadelphia: WB Saunders; 1987. p. 5.
26. Benjamin M, Curtis J. Ethics in nursing. Oxford: Oxford University Press; 1981. 95.
27. Brown JM. Conscience: the professional and the personal. J Nurs Manag 1996;4: 175–6.
28. Brody H. Conscientious objection: conflicts between personal and professional integrity. Presentation before the President's Council on Bioethics, Washington, DC, September 11, 2008.
29. Card R. Conscientious objection and emergency contraception. Am J Bioeth 2007;7(6):8–14.
30. American Nurses Association. Code of ethics with interpretive statements. 2001. Nursing World Website. Available at: http://nursingworld.org/ethics/code/protected_nwcoe813.htm. Accessed January 30, 2009.

# Art, Science, or Both? Keeping the Care in Nursing

Tayray Jasmine, PhD, MSN, RN[a,b,*]

**KEYWORDS**

• Art • Science • Nursing • Caring • Evidence-based • Research

Historically, nurses were subservient, responsive to the orders, instructions, and direction of other disciplines, specifically physicians. Physicians delegated tasks to nurses, and nurses did not necessarily question physician orders.[1] Nursing was primarily a profession of giving, and it lacked the application of scientific methodology to inform nursing practice. Nursing had not formulated formal principles of practice or evidence for procedures performed. Independent, nurse-directed regulations did not exist; autonomous decision making was limited.

In the past, the orientation of nursing was one of mother surrogate, tending and watching over a dependent ward of patients, or of a helping person. Today, laypeople often define nursing as taking care of the sick to help them get well—a definition based on media images and household ideas that is in large part a reality. The problem with this description, however, is that it limits nursing to a task-oriented, robotic duty and inaccurately depicts the complex union of art and science in nursing.[2] A definition of nursing focused on clinical hands-on functions is limiting and inconclusive. Consequently, this definition undermines the professionalization of nursing, failing to reflect its artistic and scientific foundations.

Professional nurses have now shed the handmaiden role to become caregivers on the frontlines of health care. Nursing is known as a scientific profession based on research, theory, and concepts—centered on the art of caring and focused on health care outcomes. Nursing is composed of a diverse set of practices and functions, each requiring specialized knowledge and skills. Therefore, nursing functions do not define the essence of nursing. The essence of professional nursing care is best embraced by an approach that includes its artistic and scientific dimensions.

## CARING: A THEORETICAL FRAMEWORK FOR NURSING

Through years of nursing research, caring has systematically evolved as a distinct characteristic of nursing and is now widely regarded as the theoretical framework

a Harris County Hospital District, 2525 Holly Hall, Harris County, Houston, TX 77054, USA
b Collective Healthcare Services, LLC, 2623 Sunbird Court, Pearland, TX 77584, USA
* Collective Healthcare Services, LLC, 2623 Sunbird Court, Pearland, TX 77584.
*E-mail address:* tayrayj@comcast.net

Nurs Clin N Am 44 (2009) 415–421
doi:10.1016/j.cnur.2009.07.003
0029-6465/09/$ – see front matter © 2009 Elsevier Inc. All rights reserved.

for the profession. Caring theory is an integration of common meanings in nursing that transcends settings, populations, and age groups. As a result, there are several derivatives of the meaning of nursing, all linked to and/or centered on caring. Caring is a conscious and purposeful attitude, decision, and point of reference for all behaviors and actions. Therefore, caring is an intended act resulting from conscious thought and judgment.

Caring theory rests on the assumption that humans are naturally caring to an extent and have the ability to demonstrate caring behaviors.[3] When referring to humans as naturally caring, naturally empathic is the intent. This suggests that caring is a universal value and that humans are naturally kind and concerned about others. Additionally, it is assumed that the ability to care for someone is different from possessing caring emotions. Caring is distinctly apparent when expressed—it is recognizable and observable in one's behaviors, actions, thoughts, and touch. In general, it is believed that nurses, while being naturally caring, are able to transform practice and influence each patient's caring experience with demonstrable caring behaviors and actions. Such caring behaviors are usually intangible actions, such as smiling, listening, crying, laughing, and showing interest and concern—all of which are observable.

## LINKAGE OF NURSING TO CARING

Nursing and caring are theoretically linked. Caring is the art and essence of nursing, the tradition of nursing, and the process of interaction in nursing. One may say that if you are nursing, you are caring. However, caring is more than something that nurses do; caring is something that nurses give.[4] Besides being theoretically linked to nursing, caring is an empathic exchange between the caregiver and the receiver.

Nurse researchers have explored the linkage between nursing and caring, most commonly by using a cultural, social/feminist, and/or humanistic perspective.[5] Cultural anthropologist Madeleine Leininger[6] sought to uncover the relationship between caring and cultural beliefs and also sought to learn about cultural practices and the survival of the human race. She then attempted to relate those to human health and to nursing practice.

Feminist scholar Carol Gilligan[7] sought to explain the apparent difference between the moral decision-making processes of men and those of women. She saw that a woman's basic way of being was closely related to others in the world. As a result, Gilligan speculated that women base their basic moral decision making on different foundations of caring compared with those of men.[7] Being a predominantly female profession, nursing became interested in the feminist model and research results. Since then, the model has been featured implicitly or explicitly in several nursing theories of care.

Caring theories emphasize the empathic aspects of caring, which are best defined as articulated by nursing scholar JeanWatson.[1] She describes caring as an attribute or a calling of moral commitment toward protecting human dignity and preserving humanity. Additionally, she posits that caring includes attention to and concern for the patient, individual responsibility for or providing for the patient at some level, and regard for, fondness for, or attachment to the patient.

Sara Fry,[8] a noted nurse ethicist, took the exploration of caring to another level. She suggested that researchers should move away from exploring caring along the lines of cultural, social/feminist, and humanistic models because it limits or confines the scholar to arguments and explorations that are discipline bound. She advocated a pluralistic model of caring that includes obligation and covenant formation. Fry's model combines the duty-of-care aspects with which nurses are linked—historically and bureaucratically—with the partnership and advocacy aspects of caring and with autonomy and influence that nurses aspire to in practice.[8]

## CARING: NURSE-PATIENT MUTUALITY

Nursing involves crossing one's personal barriers to thoroughly and genuinely care for another. Watson[9] refers to this as transpersonal caring, an achievement of congruency of mind, body, and spirit. This is an art in nursing that allows a nurse to move toward greater harmony with his or her mind, body, and inner soul to care for another.

Nursing and caring are grounded in a relational understanding, unity, and connection between the professional nurse and the patient. The relationship is harmonious, a give-and-take cycle of exchange. The professional nurse who is committed to caring and who has embraced caring as his or her nurse identity desires ongoing caring feedback. This feedback is used as a tool in the creation of a caring experience for the patient. The feedback is studied and applied to evidence-based research to determine the best practice for the specific patient. In turn, these caring experiences become the object of scientific inquiry.

Professional nurses are motivated and empowered by this exchange and energized to continue implementing patient-specific caring behaviors toward the goal of optimizing a patient's state of well-being. The feedback also provokes professional and personal fulfillment for nurses. Striving for fulfillment is a means that professional nurses use to care for themselves. Connecting and uniting with another individual who is in need can be draining on the professional nurse if he or she is not being fulfilled. Thus, the nurse-patient relationship embodies a shared sense of mutuality based on the patients' need and the nurses' ability. Such relationships are reciprocal in nature. For example, as a student needs a teacher, a teacher needs a student. As the teacher assists the student, the teacher is actualized and receives needed feedback from the student; the feedback promotes energy, growth, and professional and personal validation or fulfillment.

As a nurse cares for his or her patient, the nurse is actualized and receives needed fulfillment. This cycle of exchange and interconnection describes the nurse's role beyond task-oriented responsibilities. During a professional nurse's routine workday, this exchange occurs continuously with each nurse-patient interaction. As nurses enter new patient relationships or develop existing ones, he or she strives to balance a diverse set of nursing functions and caring behaviors. In achieving this balance, professional fulfillment is realized. Commitment to this balance keeps caring in nursing.

## THE SCIENCE OF NURSING: EVIDENCE-BASED PRACTICE

Professional nurses understand the importance of using the best available evidence to guide nursing practice. Those professional nurses who embrace caring as the focus of nursing possess a desire to provide safe, cost-effective, and quality nursing care by way of evidence. As opposed to intuition, good faith, or habit, the professional nurse uses evidence to make informed decisions to provide individualized patient care. This describes the process of maintaining a balance between clinical orientation and research orientation. The balance is important to professional nurses as they actively advance the scientific knowledge of nursing through research. Evidence supports nursing advancement and prevents the use of unwarranted nursing practices and nursing errors. Ultimately, evidence-based practice replaces the use of trial and error and optimizes evaluation, development, and professional advancement. Professional nurses use evidence-based practice to influence the standard of care and to promote an autonomous nursing environment.

Evidence-based practice in nursing refers to the preferential use of nursing interventions for which empiric and qualitative research has provided evidence of significant effectiveness for specific problems in nursing care. Evidence-based practice promotes the compilation, interpretation, and integration of relevant, important, and applicable patient-reported, nurse-observed, and research-driven evidence. The systematic study of theories of care and their application to patients is another example of evidence-based practice. These efforts militate against justifying nursing practice on loose bodies of knowledge—simply based on experience of other nurses—without scientific evidence on which to base nursing practice.

### THE ART OF NURSING: PERCEPTION AND THE CARING EXPERIENCE

Nursing has also been defined by the description of its clinical functions, such as maintaining or restoring normal life function, observing and reporting signs of change in a patient's condition, and assessing the patient's physical, social, and emotional state. Based on these assessments, nursing also involves formulating and performing a plan of care, counseling in relation to other health-related services and resources, and teaching to address knowledge deficits.[10] In each of these endeavors, individual patient perception is critical.

Perception is the mechanism by which an individual evaluates information received from the external environment. Cooper[11] states that perception is a critical component that precedes one's behavior and influences one's definition of certain concepts such as caring. As nurses strive to influence the caring experience of patients, individual patient perception must be understood and considered in the preparation of individualized care plans. Patient perception may present a challenge to a patient's identification of caring behaviors, as perception plays a major part in human evaluation. The results of the evaluation determine the individual's perception, which in turn influences the individual's behavioral response.

Perception is also influenced by personalities, attitudes, biases, and previous experiences. For these reasons, it is important to assess a patient's perception of caring in the planning phase of rendering caring behaviors. When a nurse knows the patient's perception of caring, he or she prepares a focused and individualized plan of care that influences the patient's caring experience.

A patient's perception of caring behaviors rendered is influenced by an interactive combination of situational, attitudinal, and behavioral biasing factors. Situational biases yield influences that affect the manner in which information is received during communication. Depending on the situation or status of the patient, caring behaviors will be accepted or rejected. The situation or status of the patient may be based on his or her perception of health and will also dictate the patient's perception of his or her need.[11] If the patient is in a situation in which he or she is diapered and soiled, verbal caring behaviors may not be perceived as caring, as he or she needs nonverbal caring behaviors, such as cleaning and/or bathing. If the patient is in a situation in which he or she is feeling discouraged and depressed, verbal caring behaviors may be needed and are accepted as caring. Professional discernment is necessary to determine whether the behaviors will be seen as caring and will successfully promote a caring experience for the patient.

Attitudinal biases include the disposition, motivation, and/or personality of the patient. Attitudinal biases also include the amount of control the patients believe they can exert on caring events. A patient's beliefs, values, and social or cultural acceptances/approvals affect his or her attitude toward caring behaviors rendered.[12] If a patient does not approve of touching because of cultural beliefs, norms, or biases, he or she may reject such nonverbal caring behaviors. In an effort to create a caring experience for patients, a professional nurse considers that an act as simple as touching may increase the patient's level of stress and be perceived as disrespectful or intrusive.

Behavioral biases are influenced by a patient's overall experience and life history. A caring expression, verbal or nonverbal, may be perceived as a risk based on the patient's history.[11] For example, a patient may respond with hostility to an attempt to comfort him physically. A routine comfort measure, such as a massage, may be perceived as a risk or an inappropriate behavior that threatens the patient's feelings of safety. As a professional nurse gets to know his or her patient, behavioral biases are assessed. Understanding a patient's behavioral biases allows nurses to successfully promote caring experiences.

## NURSING PRACTICE: CHALLENGES TO CARING

The practice of nursing is the provision of assistance to individuals or groups based on a need to maintain and/or obtain optimal health. It involves the implementation of a strategy of care or a care plan to accomplish goals set by the nurse and the individual or group. Nursing practice involves the balancing of responsibilities to the profession and to the individual receiving care. Professional nurses are accountable for giving safe and competent individualized care, guided by best practices. In providing nursing care, professional nurses are often overwhelmed by competing obligations, which, although important to the basic welfare of an individual, do not require the proficiency of a professional nurse. The arts of delegation and time management are crucial aspects, which influence the caring experience.

Performing tasks while also applying scientific concepts to care takes time. Professional nurses are often torn between the human caring model of nursing that originally attracted them to the profession and the overwhelmingly task-oriented needs and institutional demands that consume their practice time. Those professional nurses who have committed themselves to the art of caring recognize the challenge it requires and strive to maintain a balance.

In the complexity of today's health care environment, nurses are required to balance several important goals, including allocating time to anticipate caring needs, addressing priorities, establishing a trusting patient relationship, providing basic activities of living, meeting timed tasks, assessing, and evaluating. These responsibilities are challenging and may present as barriers to caring; however, a proficient professional nurse identifies those barriers and skillfully links caring behaviors in the provision of care. Accomplishing these aspects of care requires precision in understanding delegation and the need for interdisciplinary collaboration.

## THE BALANCE OF ART AND SCIENCE

The art and science of nursing are directly related to nursing autonomy and influence. Nurse autonomy is evident and supported through the profession. Professional nurses work diligently to establish and maintain an autonomous nursing environment. An autonomous nursing environment consists of a collaborative atmosphere where nursing contributions are valued, processes for participation in nursing research are established, nursing practice is refined, patient safety is assured, and caring is perceived. Self-governance thus influences nursing practice and promotes patient advocacy. Autonomous nurses are accountable and responsible to make discretionary, independent, and proactive decisions. Exercising autonomy within the confines of nursing standards of care allows nurses the opportunity to influence a patient's caring experience.

Despite barriers inherent in today's task-oriented health care environment, the professional nurse applies the art of nursing and links caring for patients as he or she takes care of patients. This describes accomplishing a harmonious balance between art and science, leading to a caring experience. The professional nurse enters a caring relationship with a patient, comes to know the patient's specific caring needs, and then demonstrates caring acts and caring behaviors to meet the patient's needs. Knowing the patient's needs is important for tailoring a nurse intervention or response. In this sense, caring requires knowledge;it is not provided based on good intention or intuition. Knowing the patient entails understanding the caring actions that are conducive to the patient's growth and well-being.[13] The caring relationship delineates a bond between the caring nurse and the patient being cared for. This bond may be referred to as an interconnection.[4]

In the profession of nursing, being interconnected means understanding the patient, viewing his or her needs as if they were the nurse's, knowing how the patient prioritizes his well-being in life, and understanding the nurse's limitations in meeting the patient's caring needs. In essence, the nurse and patient are attached and share the common goal of achieving the patient's specific and desired level of well-being. In this caring relationship, caring takes place every time the nurse-patient interaction occurs. Furthermore, care is provided in the hope of contributing to the cure or well-being of the patient. Overall, the professional nurse's goal is to care enough to make a difference in the patient's individualized sense of well-being.

## SUMMARY

Nursing is a learned and mastered art defined by the skill of anticipating the needs of others to promote health and wellness. The profession of nursing includes collective actions centered on caring.[14] The art of caring is influenced by human experience, biases, values, morals, and overall perception. Understanding that perception may serve as a barrier to one's ability to care or be cared for helps to anticipate health care outcomes. Additionally, nursing outcomes are greatly dependent on the perception of the individual receiving care. In many ways, nursing is an art and includes the proficiency of influencing perception by skillfully applying intangibles, such as empathy, kindness, compassion, solidarity, charity, and graciousness.

Science has been defined as an intellectual process for using all of one's mental and physical resources to better understand, explain, quantitate, and predict normal and unusual natural phenomena.[12] Being a system of knowledge that may be studied or learned, nursing is a science oriented to human caring, which includes arts and humanities. Nursing science includes research based on theoretical knowledge that is reflective, subjective, objective, and interpretive.[14]

Professional nurses are accountable for the influence they have on a patient's perception of care. This influence should not be taken for granted and includes the art of causing an effect in an intangible caring way. Nurses further influence the caring experience and health care outcome of patients by applying evidence-based research to nursing practice.

The scientific knowledge that supports nursing and caring has been studied, observed, researched, and tested. Though the words *nursing* and *caring* are often used synonymously, the acts are unique, as nursing is an art and a science, and caring is the art and science that defines nursing.

**REFERENCES**

1. Watson J. Nursing: a science and human care. Norwalk (CT): Appleton Century Crofts; 1985.
2. Allmark P. Is caring a virtue? J Adv Nurs 1998;28(3):466–73.
3. Boykin A, Schoenhofer S. Nursing as caring: a model for transforming practice. Massachusetts: Jones and Bartlett Publishers; 2001.
4. Watson J, Foster R. The attending nurse caring model: integrating theory, evidence and advanced caring-healing therapeutics for transforming professional practice. J Clin Nurs 2003;12(3):360–6.
5. Wilkes L, Wallis M. A model of professional nurse caring: nursing students' experience. J Adv Nurs 1998;27(3):582–90.
6. Leininger M. Transcultural care diversity and university: a theory of nursing. New Jersey: Charles B. Slack; 1985.
7. Gilligan C. In a different voice: psychological theory and women's development. Cambridge: Harvard University Press; 1982.
8. Fry S. Research on ethics in nursing: the state of the art. Nurs Outlook 1987;35(5): 256.
9. Watson J. Nursing: human science and human care: a theory of nursing. New York: National League for Nursing; 1988.
10. Kelly L. The nursing experience: trends, challenges, and transitions. 2nd edition. New York: McGraw Hill, Inc. 1992.
11. Cooper D. Psychology, risk, and safety: understanding how personality and perception can influence risk taking. Prof Saf 2003;48(11):39–46.
12. Thomas C. Taber's cyclopedic medical dictionary. 16th edition. Philadelphia: F.A. Davis Company; 1989.
13. Mayeroff M. On caring. New York: Harper and Row Publishers; 1971.
14. Watson J, Smith M. Caring science and the science of unitary human beings: a trans-theoretical discourse for nursing knowledge development. J Adv Nurs 2002;37(5):452–62.

# Moral Accountability and Integrity in Nursing Practice

Cynthia Ann LaSala, MS, RN[a,b,*]

**KEYWORDS**

- Ethics • Nursing • Moral accountability • Integrity
- Moral agency

## HISTORICAL PERSPECTIVE

Florence Nightingale believed that nursing was a calling and that the work of nursing focused on health restoration, health promotion, and disease prevention. She identified healing as central to the practice of nursing, and leadership and global action as the basis for advancing the health of individuals and communities. Nightingale stressed the importance of accountability, consistency, and truthfulness in practice. She maintained that the nurse's ability to form therapeutic relationships was predicated on caring, healing, and clarity of purpose. Nurses were to consider themselves role models, maintaining dignity and presence in their interactions with patients, families, and one another and being personally responsible for their moral conduct.

Nightingale envisioned nursing as an art and a science, a "calling," and an interpersonal process of caring and healing across life's continuum.[1] As an early progenitor of feminist theory about caring, she promoted an ethic of caring and healing among nurses as a way of maintaining wholeness, and she perceived the nurse's ability to care for his or her self as an essential component. Caring for oneself enables the person to be more compassionate, kind, merciful, gentle, and giving toward others. She believed that a nurse achieves "the moral ideal" whenever he or she uses "the whole self" to form relationships with "the whole of the person receiving care."[1] She described knowing what is right and wrong as "inward values" and advocated for integrating ethical decision making and personal accountability for one's own moral behavior into professional practice.[1] In her reflections on nurses as leaders, Nightingale embraced the concept of moral accountability: "Let whoever is in charge keep this simple question in her head (*not*, how can I always do this right thing myself, *but*) how can I provide for this right thing to be done?"[2]

[a] Department of Nursing, Massachusetts General Hospital, 55 Fruit Street, Boston, MA 02114, USA
[b] The American Nurses Association Center for Ethics and Human Rights, 8515 Georgia Avenue, Suite 400, Silver Spring, MD 20910, USA
* Massachusetts General Hospital, 55 Fruit Street, Boston, MA 02114.
*E-mail address:* clasala@partners.org

Nurs Clin N Am 44 (2009) 423–434
doi:10.1016/j.cnur.2009.07.006
0029-6465/09/$ – see front matter

Despite the current realities that challenge nursing accountability, integrity, and responsibility in practice, Nightingale's work as reflected in her writings and observations laid the groundwork for the evolution of nursing into a trusted profession. To be morally accountable is to appropriately defend and substantiate one's decisions based on moral values and norms.[3] Nightingale challenges us to know and to do what is right to further the cause of quality patient care, duty to self, and duty to others: "We should strive for what we can best do and what is most attractive and thereby find 'our duty'."[2]

The American Nurses Association (ANA) *Code of Ethics for Nurses* clearly articulates what society should expect from nurses and the community of nursing at large in terms of professional practice. Nurses are guided by scope and standards of practice in their decision making concerning an appropriate course of action to which they are accountable (answerable) and responsible. Nurses who are morally accountable make informed, reasonable judgments based on what is right, and they act accordingly. Having integrity "includes wholeness of character, attention to one's own welfare or self- care, and emotional integrity reliant on maintaining relational boundaries."[4]

## NURSING PRACTICE AND THE ETHIC OF CARING

Nurses affect the lives of young and old, from birth to end of life, in profound and unique ways. What is the basis for this call to service? Why do patients identify nurses as central to their recovery in achieving or regaining an optimal level of wellness? What sustains nurses in their practice?

Jean Watson,[5] a preeminent scholar of care theory in nursing, states that "the caring moment can be an existential turning point for the nurse, in that it involves pausing, choosing to "see"; it is informed action guided by an intentionality and consciousness of how to *be* in the moment—fully present…" The nurse grows in his or her understanding of what it means to be more human by connecting with the patient and others in a way that facilitates a "wisdom in knowing"—an increased capacity to show compassion and care through a sense of shared humanity.[5] It is through this self-awareness that the nurse begins to see caring in a deeper sense, which embodies Nightingale's concept of nursing as a "calling" and a commitment to compassionate and loving service predicated on a value system that is humanistic and concerned with the welfare of others.[5]

In discussing her Caring Science model, Watson[5] asserts that a "caring consciousness" assists patients in connecting with their internal potential to heal while preserving the "human dignity, wholeness, and integrity" of the person. The quality and effectiveness of the caring relationship between the patient and the nurse is largely dependent on the nurse's willingness and "ability to be authentically present in a way that reaches out to the other," which Watson describes as "the transpersonal nature" of this relationship.[5] The transpersonal "*Caritas Consciousness* nurse" sees beyond what may be immediately apparent. He or she is more alert to the here and now and to the nuances of the patient's situation and uses "empiric-technical, ethical, intuitive, personal, aesthetic, even spiritual knowing."[5] This nurse has a deeper sense of satisfaction, becomes centered, and is more precise in his or her assessments, which enhances the nurse-patient relationship. Watson[5] describes *Caritas Consciousness* as "a professional ideal to guide one's moral and ethical commitment and intentionality with each patient and sustain nursing's caring mission and covenant with society." Watson[5] submits that "a caring attitude" is not something that is genetically passed on from one generation to the next but rather through "the culture of society." She refers to "the discipline and profession of nursing" as "the culture of nursing" and the pivotal role nurses play through the art and science of nursing in "advancing, sustaining, and preserving human caring" in fulfilling their covenant with society and humanity.[5]

## CASE STUDY: TO KNOW

Consider the experience of a registered nurse, practicing on a general medical and oncology unit, who shares her insights in this excerpt from a narrative that she wrote about caring for a 40-year-old woman with non-Hodgkin lymphoma who was admitted with a hematocrit value of 16 after her first cycle of chemotherapy treatment as an outpatient. The patient was a Jehovah's Witness and clearly stated that she did not want to be transfused blood, based on her religious beliefs.

> "JD arrived on the floor...As she sat on the bed I looked at her with a concerned expression and she said, "Don't ask me about the blood transfusion. I will be fine. God is watching over me." I nodded my head and respected her wishes. Over the next several days, JD's hematocrit wavered from 16 to 18. As her doctors hovered over possible alternatives to blood transfusions, JD sat in her room comfortably surrounded by her family. Also of concern was her growing tumor burden from her lymphoma. Her attending physician...when speaking with her hematologist...said, "This is ridiculous. She should just take some blood and it would solve so many of her problems. I don't even know why Jehovahs refuse blood." I explained to him what her beliefs were and why she refused blood. He continued to look confused and I said, "We may not understand it fully, but we have to respect her decision and not let our personal opinions impede our care." He looked at me and said I was absolutely right." (Courtesy of Lindsay O'Brien, RN, BSN, Boston, MA.)

This narrative illustrates the nurse's ability to form a trusting and caring relationship with her patient by acknowledging the wholeness of the person as a critical element in clinical decision making. The nurse-patient relationship is central to the ethic of caring. In the context of this relationship, the nurse is accountable "to act under a code of ethical conduct that is grounded in the moral principles of fidelity and respect for the dignity, worth, and self-determination of patients."[6] Moreover, as Olson[7] suggests, the nurse's moral character is expressed in "who we are and what we do, even when no one else sees."

## BARRIERS TO CARING PRACTICES

Nursing continues to struggle with defining itself as an art and a science, requiring enormous skill and a unique body of knowledge that is firmly grounded in caring practice. In many instances, market forces and cost-containment measures have attempted to minimize the complexities of practice and the critical role that the nurse-patient relationship plays in effecting a therapeutic, caring environment that meets the physiologic and psychosocial needs of the patient. Is it one's role or how one operationalizes it that brings together the knowledge, skill, and caring practice characteristic of professional nursing? Harrison[8] asks, "What does the concept of 'caring' really mean, and what can be done to remove barriers to caring in nursing practice?"

On completion of orientation (which focuses on acquisition of job-related competencies to meet role expectations), novice nurses frequently describe a sense of being left on their own to negotiate the difficult transition from novice to professional nurse. One Nevada study revealed a 30% attrition rate among 352 new registered nurses in the first year and 57% in the second year because of the difficult realities of role transition (ie, staffing shortages, increased acuity, unacceptable patient to nurse ratios, decreased support and guidance, management issues).[9] Findings from another study of 843 nurses suggest that younger nurses experience higher levels of stress, agitation, and burnout.[10]

Surveys suggest that the demands of care and the lack of adequate resources to safely provide an appropriate level of care are resulting in nurses leaving not only their positions but also their profession. Hayes and Scott[11] reported that a 20% vacancy rate among registered nurses is expected by 2010 and is currently estimated at 14% nationwide. Factors that contribute to the turnover among novice nurses include short staffing, stress associated with increased workload and patient acuity, inadequate leadership support, level of responsibility, and practice in environments that compromise quality care and safe practice. Granger[12] reported that the National Sample Survey of Registered Nurses in March 2000 demonstrated that 44.9% of registered nurses who have professions other than nursing consider those professions more rewarding than their nursing positions. Further illustrating this issue is a US Department of Health and Human Services report that documents a 28% increase in the number of registered nurses unemployed in nursing.[12]

The advancement of professional nursing depends on the ability to develop nursing leaders who will work toward unity within the profession and guide, direct, and advocate for change that will promote professional competence and personal growth. Competency in caring must be regarded as an essential component of professional practice in addition to the psychomotor and cognitive skills that are required. However, the caring in health care can become obscured by an emphasis on getting the job done, technological advances, and economics rather than embracing caring practices and building caring relationships at the point of care. Systems and work environments must direct their efforts toward actively engaging nurses in decision making at unit and organizational levels, promoting autonomy in practice, and identifying strategies for implementing and sustaining an ethic of care. Nightingale's words hold true today as they did when she addressed the Congress on Hospitals, Dispensaries, and Nursing at the World's Fair in Chicago in 1893:

> "No system can endure that does not march. Are we walking to the future or to the past? Are we progressing or are we stereotyping? We remember that we have scarcely crossed the threshold of uncivilized civilization in nursing: there is still so much to do. Don't let us stereotype mediocrity. We are still on the threshold of nursing."[2]

## CASE STUDY: TO REASON

Boykin and colleagues[13] reported about a research project that was conducted on an 18-bed telemetry unit at a 350-bed for-profit hospital in Atlantis, Florida. The purpose of the project was to illustrate how implementation of a caring practice model using the theory of Nursing as Caring and a key element, the "Dance of Caring Persons," could potentially increase patient-nurse satisfaction and institutional recognition as a provider of quality health care.[13]

Staff in direct or indirect patient care roles were asked to share stories that demonstrated caring practice, described the nature of the caring practice relevant to the situation, characterized the experience as caring, and exemplified key components of quality health care. An analysis of these data identified several themes: commitment; a desire to be present based on concern for others; the ability to know and respond to what is important, which is contingent upon listening; caring practice that nurtures individuals through the caring experience; a sense of value from the shared experience; and valuing the contributions of the interdisciplinary team.[13]

Staff were then asked to identify strategies for redesigning the practice model, which would incorporate what they valued most. Strategies included a visual display and brief narratives about individual staff members to help patients, families, and staff know about the person who was providing care. Other interventions included a unit-based library of literature related to caring in nursing and sharing personal and professional practice stories. To enhance communication and to meet patients' and families' priorities, new patients were given a greeting card with the number to the nurses' station and a pad of paper and pen so that they could record questions. Lastly, the staff suggested creating flexible work schedules to better accommodate the needs of the staff and provide appropriate staffing, and redesigning the performance appraisal system to more accurately reflect caring values.[13]

Staff used "direct invitation"[13] to promote meaningful dialog between patients, families, and one another to identify priorities of care and the essence of caring practice. A computerized database was created to document patient and family requests that informed unit practice among nurses and members of the interdisciplinary team. Nurses became less focused on the tasks at hand and more aware of the caring nature of their peers and administrative staff, which transformed the work environment. Teambuilding was enhanced, and the caring practice model that was adopted became a positive recruitment and retention tool.[13]

What was learned as a result of this project? Clearly that practice can be transformed through a renewed understanding of the basic values germane to nursing and the development of new ways for interrelating with patients, families, peers, and at the organizational level. The nurses' commitment to the values and beliefs that were personally and professionally most important to them promoted positive change within the workplace. Watson[5] speaks about the importance of creating a healing environment in practice, whereby "wholeness, beauty, comfort, and peace" may be realized. Provision 6 of the ANA *Code of Ethics for Nurses* states that "the nurse participates in establishing, maintaining, and improving health care environments and conditions of employment conducive to the provision of quality health care and consistent with the values of the profession through individual and collective action."[6]

The core values of human dignity, respect, caring, and compassion are not only central to the care of patients but also to nurses' interactions with one another, members of the interdisciplinary team, and others. Nurses, as key players in an organization's culture, mission, and goals, are empowered to be accountable in their practice and create meaningful change when they are treated equitably and respectfully and are genuinely embraced by leadership.[7] It is through a sense of shared accountability that nurses recognize the inherent worth and contributions of those with whom they work, which promotes job satisfaction and the development of cohesive teams.[14] Through this project, patient and staff satisfaction was enhanced by rethinking and recreating the nursing practice model to achieve identified goals and a shared vision.[13]

## MORAL AND LEGAL ACCOUNTABILITY IN NURSING PRACTICE

*Nursing's Social Policy Statement* provides professional nurses with a framework for understanding their covenant with society and obligation to those entrusted to their care. This document describes what professional nursing is, its scope of practice, knowledge base, and methods for regulation of the profession. In this document, nursing is defined as "the protection, promotion, and optimization of health and

not include a permission to practice poorly; it presupposes an obligation to practice well."

## WHAT IS MORAL AGENCY?

In an editorial that appeared in *Nursing Outlook* in 1999, Hamric[23] posed the question, "What does it mean to say that professional nurses are moral agents?" The answer to this question lies in the ANA *Code of Ethics for Nurses*, which identifies the nurse's commitment to provide safe, competent care and advocate for patients as fundamental to professional practice. Being morally accountable and responsible for one's judgment and actions is central to the nurse's role as a moral agent. The reality of the current health care environment challenges the nurse's ability to exercise moral agency in confronting the bureaucracy and depersonalization that can occur in the work setting. Research has demonstrated that a nurse's willingness to act in addressing ethical dilemmas in practice is contingent on 4 factors: level of clinical expertise, the degree to which nurses perceive themselves as influential in their respective work environments, demonstrated interest or concern for ethical issues, and a knowledge base in ethics.[23]

Bishop and Scudder[24] suggest that a "morally good" nurse uses his or her skills to effect safe, competent care. Nurses practice in the best interest of the patients, which implies that the nurse's interventions are intrinsically moral. Nurses take risks and act with moral courage in the face of uncertainty when the situation demands it to promote and preserve the well-being of the patient.[24] In a study that explored the influence of the work environment on nurses' health, "morally habitable environments" were defined as "those that foster recognition, cooperation, and the shared benefit of many goods, as opposed to those that engender oppression, suffering, deception, and violence."[25] Nurses across all settings and roles share accountability for adopting a professional value system, identifying and implementing changes that will improve the practice environment and maintaining competency. The concepts of moral accountability and responsibility are essential to human dignity.[14] Holding oneself and one's colleagues accountable has been identified as a key component for ethical competence among health care professionals.[26]

## WHAT IS MORAL INTEGRITY AS A PERSONAL AND PROFESSIONAL VALUE?

What does possessing integrity really mean? How does having moral integrity as a nurse relate to knowing and acting in an ethical manner? Is it possible for nurses to maintain their moral integrity in a health care climate replete with constant change, fiscal constraint, shifting leadership, staffing shortages, and a seemingly vacillating value system? Are the risks to nurses' moral integrity and the ramifications of those risks issues that the nursing profession and the health care industry are prepared to address? Can we afford not to?

Possessing integrity implies having a sense of unity—of that which is complete and whole.[27] Integrity encompasses one's personal values and involves maintaining a healthy equilibrium between physical, psychosocial, and intellectual concerns. Integrity also includes autonomy. An individual's self-determination may be diminished or disrespected when one's integrity is threatened or violated. One's value system forms the basis for personal integrity, whereas moral integrity is predicated on mutually accepted ethical standards and principles.[27] Nurses who respect the uniqueness of each patient and engage the patient in shared decision making and self-care safeguard the patient's integrity when he or she is rendered most vulnerable by illness and disease. The moral integrity of the nurse is critical to the patient's personal integrity.[27]

Integrity has also been defined as "a deeply personal phenomenon" and "the correlation between actions on the one hand and beliefs, principles, or convictions on the other."[28] A nurse who withholds administering a medication to a patient because of safety concerns and a commitment to do no harm acts with moral integrity. A sense of oneself or personal identity (self-understanding) informs one's actions—that which an individual understands is the right thing to do is consistent with that which he or she does.[28]

## CASE STUDY: THE ETHIC OF CARE

The relationship that the nurse forms with the patient is the "moral center of nursing practice."[29] Listen to the words of a novice nurse as she recounts her experience in caring for a 40-year-old patient admitted with pancytopenia, fever, and cellulitis of his left arm after chemotherapy treatment for acute myelocytic leukemia:

> *"In my practice as a nurse I feel that with each patient you learn something new, but it's not from every patient that you take something away. MC and I had a great clinical relationship. I learned a lot from his complex clinical case and at times had to admit that I didn't have the answers to his questions. MC made me feel so comfortable that I was not afraid to tell him that I didn't always have the answers. MC taught me a lot about courage and taking each day as it comes. He met each challenge with a smile and helped me to feel confident as a new nurse...MC had mentioned me as one of his "best nurses." For the first time as a nurse I felt that I was in the right place and doing the right thing." (Courtesy of Brianna Antle, RN, BSN, Boston, MA.)*

Decisions regarding doing what is morally acceptable frequently involve more than one person or party. As a patient advocate, the nurse is in a unique position to build consensus, promote interdisciplinary collaboration, and positively influence outcomes that would support rather than oppose moral decision making among members of the health care team.[30] During times of uncertainty, increased vulnerability, and hopelessness, nurses must renew their commitment to learn more and to reassess personal values and their sense of purpose in their work with patients, families, other disciplines, and one another. In doing so, nurses promote and sustain a caring, healing practice in their interactions with others and themselves.

Hamric[30] refers to instances where the personal and/or professional values of a nurse are in conflict with what is right and just as "being in-the-middle," which may predispose the nurse to moral distress, burnout, loss of integrity, and significant conflict. The nurse may feel alienated, increasingly vulnerable, and powerless in his or her attempt to find a solution that is in concert with personal values, beliefs, obligations, and moral integrity. Veneta Masson,[31] a nurse, poet, and essayist, described an experience in her practice while caring for a poverty-stricken, bedridden, elderly woman living by herself in a community plagued by drug dealers and users. She recounts how she was pressured by other health professionals to stop caring for this patient, so as to induce a crisis that would allow the city to intervene and to force the patient "into a nursing home where she belonged." The patient was steadfast in her determination to remain in her own home until "...the Lord called her. Not before." Masson engaged in reflective practice through journaling, which enabled her to better understand her patient's needs, to be present, and to establish a therapeutic, caring relationship with her patient. She refers to the art of nursing manifested in her poetry as self-sustaining to her practice and the reason why she chose the nursing profession.

She describes "the heart of nursing" as being "the art of nursing"[31] and perceives this art as a powerful tool to unify, sustain, and advance the profession. Hamric suggests that the concept of fidelity (remaining faithful to one's personal and professional commitments and promises), as illustrated by Masson's story, can serve as a useful framework for better understanding the ethical nature of "being in-the-middle" and may offer nurses opportunities that help to preserve their moral integrity and to promote moral decision making.[30]

## NURSING'S COVENANT

Nursing demonstrates a commitment to its covenant with society and the advancement of the profession when nurses provide care to patients based on the goals, values, and integrity inherent in nursing practice.[32] Provision 5 of the ANA *Code of Ethics for Nurses* states that "the nurse owes the same duties to self as to others, including the responsibility to preserve integrity and safety, to maintain competence, and to continue personal and professional growth."[6] The *Code* clearly states that nurses are obligated to consistently maintain their personal and professional values when responding to situations that challenge their moral integrity and to accept compromise "only to the degree that it remains an integrity-preserving compromise."[6]

Although nurses across all settings and roles may conscientiously object (refuse to participate) in instances that directly oppose their personal and/or professional moral standards and may endanger patients, abandoning a patient is never morally acceptable. The nurse must communicate, as soon as possible, his or her decision to withdraw from care or to refuse to provide a specific treatment, to assure the appropriate transfer of care. Although these actions may not protect nurses from incurring the consequences, legal or otherwise, conscientious objection does allow nurses to maintain their moral integrity in their refusal to participate in activities or interventions they deem unacceptable.[6]

Nurses are morally obligated to report inappropriate practice or behavior in their work environments that place the patient's or nurse's well-being at risk and to serve as catalysts for change to resolve these issues.[6] The nurse's first commitment has always been to the patient. However, nurses are also morally obligated to maintain their fidelity in their interactions with families and facilitate outcomes that support rather than oppose moral decision making among members of the health care team.[30] Practicing with integrity involves acting consistently and with self-understanding.[28] The nurse who is mindful and observant of the challenges inherent in caring recognizes self-understanding as essential to maintaining personal integrity.

## SUMMARY

The exemplars of the art and science of professional nursing are compassionate caring, moral accountability, and integrity. Despite the inherent challenges, nurses remain committed to making a difference in people's lives, and in doing so, they find joy and personal satisfaction in giving of themselves in service to others while being personally and professionally transformed by the experience.

Nightingale inspires us to renew our commitment to remaining steadfast in this journey:

> *"Let us be anxious to do well, not for selfish praise but to honor and advance the cause, the work we have taken up. Let us value our training not as it makes us cleverer or superior to others, but inasmuch as it enables us to be more useful and helpful to our fellow creatures, the sick, who most want our help. Let it be our*

*ambition to be…good nurses, and never let us be ashamed of the name of 'nurse'.*"[2]

The light from Nightingale's lamp continues to be a beacon of hope, inspiration, and healing for all those who are entrusted to nurses' care, and may it provide a source of renewal, wisdom, and strength for the future of professional nursing practice.

## ACKNOWLEDGMENT

Many individuals have influenced and inspired my professional practice and career in nursing. My colleague and mentor, Ellen Robinson, RN, PhD, Clinical Nurse Specialist in Ethics at Massachusetts General Hospital, has cultivated my knowledge base and love of ethics and assisted me in identifying my approach to this project. To Lindsay, Alexis, and Brianna and the many highly committed nurses in the past and present who I have been privileged to interface with and learn from in my daily practice…you are shining examples of moral accountability, moral integrity, and caring presence that is lived. The Nightingale legacy of caring, compassionate service, healing, advocacy, and leadership continues…

## REFERENCES

1. Dossey BM, Selanders LC, Beck DM, et al. Florence Nightingale's 13 formal letters to her nurses (1872–1900). In: Florence Nightingale today: healing, leadership, global action. Silver Spring (MD): American Nurses Association; 2005. p. 49, 52–3.
2. Ulrich BT. Leadership. In: Leadership and management according to Florence Nightingale. Norwalk (CT): Appleton & Lange; 1992. p. 43, 54, 11, 111.
3. Badzek LA. Provision four. In: Fowler MDM, editor. Guide to the code of ethics for nurses: interpretation and application. Silver Spring (MD): Nursebooks.org; 2008. p. 43–5.
4. Fowler MDM. Provision five. In: Fowler MDM, editor. Guide to the code of ethics for nurses: interpretation and application. Silver Spring (MD): Nursebooks.org; 2008. p. 58.
5. Watson J. In nursing: the philosophy and science of caring. Boulder (CO): University Press of Colorado; 2008. p. 5, 91, 77–9, 82, 18, 31.
6. American Nurses Association. Code of ethics for nurses with interpretive statements. Silver Spring (MD): American Nurses Publishing; 2001. p. 16, 18–20.
7. Olson LL. Provision six. In: Fowler MDM, editor. Guide to the code of ethics for nurses: interpretation and application. Silver Spring (MD): Nursebooks.org; 2008. p. 76, 74.
8. Harrison LL. Maintaining the ethic of caring in nursing. J Adv Nurs 2006;54(3): 255–7.
9. Bowles C, Candela L. First job experiences of recent RN graduates: improving the work environment. J Nurs Adm 2005;35(3):130–7.
10. Erickson RJ, Grove WC. Why emotions matter: age, agitation, and burnout among registered nurses. Online J Issues Nurs 2001;6(1). Availble at:http://www.nursingworld.org/MainMenuCategories/ANAMarketplace/ANAPeriodicals/O. Accessed December 28, 2008.
11. Hayes JM, Scott AS. Mentoring partnerships as the wave of the future for new graduates. Nurs Educ Perspect 2007;28(1):27–9.

12. Granger TA. Mentoring: leading the way toward positive change. Sigma Theta Tau International Web site. Available at: http://nursingsociety.org/RNL/3Q-2006/features/features8.html?type=print. Accessed December 27, 2008.

13. Boykin A, Schoenhofer SO, Smith N, et al. Transforming practice using a caring-based nursing model. Nurs Adm Q 2003;27(3):223–30.

14. Kupperschmidt BR. Making a case for shared accountability. J Nurs Adm 2004; 34(3):114–6.

15. American Nurses Association. Nursing's social policy statement. 2nd edition. Washington, DC: American Nurses Publishing; 2003. p. 6, 11.

16. American Nurses Association. Principles for delegation. Silver Spring (MD): American Nurses Association; 2005. p. 4.

17. Bishop AH, Scudder JR Jr. Nursing ethics: holistic caring practice. 2nd edition. Sudbury (MA): Jones and Bartlett; 2001. p. 128–9.

18. Muyskens JL. The nurse as a member of a profession. In: Pence T, Cantrall J, editors. Ethics in nursing: an anthology. New York: National League for Nursing; 1990. p. 288–90. Pub. No. 20-2294.

19. Hamric AB. What is happening to advocacy? Nurs Outlook 2000;48(3):103–4.

20. Fry ST. Philosophical and theoretical issues in nursing ethics. In: Pinch WJE, Haddad AM, editors. Nursing and health care ethics: a legacy and a vision. Silver Spring (MD): Nursebooks.org; 2008. p. 51–3.

21. Hayes C. Linking Newman's theory of health as expanding consciousness to ethics and caring. In: Picard C, Jones D, editors. Giving voice to what we know: Margaret Newman's theory of health as expanding consciousness in nursing practice, research, and education. Sudbury (MA): Jones and Bartlett; 2005. p. 29.

22. Curtin L. The commitment of nursing. In: Pence T, Cantrall J, editors. Ethics in nursing: an anthology. New York: National League for Nursing; 1990. p. 284. Pub. No. 20-2294.

23. Hamric AB. The nurse as moral agent in modern health care. Nurs Outlook 1999; 47(3):106.

24. Bishop AH, Scudder JR Jr. The primacy of caring practice in nursing ethics. In: Pinch WJE, Haddad AM, editors. Nursing and health care ethics: a legacy and a vision. Silver Spring (MD): Nursebooks.org; 2008. p. 216–9.

25. Peter EH, MacFarlane AV, O'Brien-Pallas LL. Analysis of the moral habitability of the nursing work environment. J Adv Nurs 2004;47(4):356–64.

26. Taylor CR. Right relationships: foundation for health care ethics. In: Pinch WJE, Haddad AM, editors. Nursing and health care ethics: a legacy and a vision. Silver Spring (MD): Nursebooks.org; 2008. p. 163.

27. Widang I, Fridlund B. Self-respect, dignity and confidence: conceptions of integrity among male patients. J Adv Nurs 2003;42(1):47–56.

28. Moland LL. Moral integrity and regret in nursing. In: Nelson S, Gordon S, editors. The complexities of care – nursing reconsidered. Ithaca (NY): ILR/Cornell University Press; 2006. p. 52, 67.

29. D'Antonio P. Nursing and health care ethics: a legacy. In: Pinch WJE, Haddad AM, editors. Nursing and health care ethics: a legacy and a vision. Silver Spring (MD): Nursebooks.org; 2008. p. 11.

30. Hamric AB. Reflections on being in the middle. Nurs Outlook 2001;49(6):254–7.

31. Masson V. Ninth street notebook: voice of a nurse in the city. Washington, DC: Sage Femme Press; 2001. p. 124–6.

32. American Nurses Association. Nursing: scope and standards of practice. Washington, DC: Nursebooks.org; 2001. p.18.

# Nursing Advocacy in a Postgenomic Age

Rebekah Hamilton, PhD, RN

**KEYWORDS**

- Ethics • Genetics • Genomics • Nursing advocacy
- Nursing competencies

## NURSING AND GENETICS

The study of genetics and genomics is increasingly considered an essential science for all areas of health care,[1] requiring skill in risk assessment, genetic testing, diagnosis, targeted prevention strategies, pharmacogenomics, and genetic therapies.[2] Although nurses must be knowledgeable of the science of genetics and have skills to engage patients, they must also understand the complexities that may arise for individuals and families. This ability to reason beyond just the clinical science and consider the wider implications of genomic health care will allow the nurse to be a true patient advocate. To reason may mean to assist the patient and family in understanding the ramifications of a genetic diagnosis, communicate the meaning of a test result, and empathize with the potential implications of new genetic knowledge. In addition, practicing in this era also requires an ethical sensitivity to the new issues raised by genomic health care.

Like most health care professionals, nurses are faced with a wealth of new information on genetics in disease and health. The average age of nurses in the United States is 47 years, and 41% of registered nurses (RNs) are 50 years or older, with only 8% less than the age of 30 years.[3] It is likely that most RNs have received little, if any, genetics education since the completion of the first phase of the Human Genome Project in 2003. The Human Genome Project was a successful international effort to sequence and map the entire human genome.[4] Professional nursing and medical organizations have attempted to address this need. The International Society of Nurses in Genetics (ISONG) was formed in 1988 with 83 members[5] and now has more than 400 members from 14 countries. The role of this organization is to foster the scientific and professional growth of nurses in human genetics and genomics worldwide.[6]

In 1995, the American Nurses Association (ANA) addressed the issue of the nurse's role in managing genetic information, discussing informed consent, truth telling, confidentiality, and nondiscrimination.[7] In 1996, the American Medical Association (AMA),

Department of Women, Children and Family Health Science (MC 802), College of Nursing, University of Illinois at Chicago, 845 South Damen Avenue, Chicago, IL 60612, USA
*E-mail address:* hamilr@uic.edu

Nurs Clin N Am 44 (2009) 435–446
doi:10.1016/j.cnur.2009.07.007
0029-6465/09/$ – see front matter © 2009 Elsevier Inc. All rights reserved.

the ANA, and the National Human Genome Research Institute (NHGRI) of the National Institutes of Health (NIH) formed the collaborative "organization of organizations" committed to promoting health care professional education in human genetics, the National Coalition for Health Professional Education in Genetics (NCHPEG).[8]

In 2004 in the United States, an effort was begun by NHGRI and the National Cancer Institute (NCI) to establish the essential nursing competencies for genetics and genomics. This effort resulted in a list of essential competencies applying to all RNs, "with the expectation that competent nursing practice now requires the incorporation of genetic and genomic knowledge and skills."[9] The update of *The Essentials of Baccalaureate Education for Professional Nursing Practice* by the American Association of Colleges of Nursing (AACN)[10] recommends that genomic content be included in the nursing curriculum as one of the foundational sciences, in areas of clinical prevention and population health, as an area for continuous self-evaluation and lifelong learning, and as a component of the Bachelor of Science Generalist Nursing curriculum.

One example of a nursing organization that has embraced the importance of genetics to practice is the Oncology Nursing Society (ONS). ONS offers online updates, regional classes, and position statements relative to genetics (http://www.ons.org/). As the specialty of oncology has moved ahead in prediction, diagnosis, and treatment of cancers by implementing genetic testing, tumor marker testing, and chemotherapy designed specifically for the tumor type, oncology nurses have stayed abreast of these genetic developments.

Efforts at nursing education in genetics are not limited to the United States. For example, in 2004, the International Council of Nurses (ICN) published a monograph on various topics of importance about genetics in nursing and described the activities of nurses in genetics in several countries.[11]

In looking at nursing's role in the implementation and advancement of patient care in the era of genomic health care, this special issue addresses the following topics "What do nurses need to know about genetics?" "What does it mean to reason relative to genetics?" and "When to act and what to do?" Although a significant number of RNs are updating this knowledge of genetics and genomics, it must be argued that knowledge of the science and the broader ethical, legal, and social issues is essential in this postgenomic age.[5] This discussion is organized to address the general categories of knowing, reasoning, and acting, as conceptualized in this special issue. Each of these categories has been used as an exemplar of how nursing and genetics come together in practice.

**WHAT TO KNOW**

Knowledge is the basis of understanding, and in nursing, the foundation of practice. Knowledge begins with basic understanding of terminology. Although these are complex concepts, in this article genetics is defined as the study of individual genes and their effect on rare single-gene disorders. Genomics is defined as the study of all the genes in the human genome together, including their interactions with each other, the environment, and the influence of other psychosocial and cultural factors.[12]

Knowledge of genetics and genomics includes understanding the implications of its significance in patients' lives, thus the meaning of genomics in health is a critical aspect of nursing practice. With any disease mechanism, it is important for nurses to have knowledge of the underlying physiologic and molecular processes, for such a foundation forms the basis of clinical reasoning. Understanding the genetic component of diseases requires knowledge of fundamental genetic science.[8] Examples of basic genetic information include:

- Genetics at the molecular level: DNA and RNA replication, types of mutations, and so on
- Genetics behind human diversity: definition of polymorphism and understanding of how small gene changes affect diversity
- Types of genetic disorders: single-gene and complex disorders
- Interactions of the environment and genetic expression: finding genetic factors that influence the risks for diabetes, cancer, high blood pressure, and other common disorders
- Types of genetic testing: carrier, prenatal, newborn, presymptomatic, and diagnostic
- Prevention and treatment of genetic diseases: gene therapies, pharmacogenomics, targeted treatments.[13]

These examples of expected nursing competency correspond to the knowledge, understanding, and expertise needed by nurses in a postgenomic age. Practicing in this era also requires an ethical sensitivity to the new issues raised by genomic health care.

## HOW TO REASON

Integral to competent nursing practice is the ability to go beyond the scientific knowledge of genomics and examine the larger implications of genomics in health care. It is critical that nurses understand the ethical, legal, and social implications that arise when genomics becomes part of health care practice. From the early start of the Human Genome Project, leaders in the field understood the importance of genetic advances and the impact on individuals, families, communities and cultures, and society.[14] Scholars continue to explore issues such as discrimination based on genetic risk, ownership of DNA, patenting of genes, and informed consent as greater understanding of the role of genes in health is discovered.[15] Examples of how nurses can use critical thinking and reasoning skills in prenatal, diagnostic, and presymptomatic genetic testing are discussed in the following sections.

### Prenatal Genetic Testing

Most nurses are familiar with prenatal genetics because nursing curricula have typically addressed topics such as chromosomal anomalies, metabolic disorders, and environmental mutagens (eg, thalidomide). However, as knowledge of genetic mutations and associated disease risks increase, what may be less understood are the growing implications of prenatal genetic testing. More than 1600 disease-associated mutations have been identified, (http://www.genetests.org/) providing information about the risk for and/or diagnosis of a given disease.

Although most people agree that adults may decide to have genetic testing to evaluate their risk for passing on a potentially harmful mutation to their offspring, the disability community and others have raised questions about an expansion of prenatal testing.[16] This difficult area was examined by a group of professionals interested in disability issues and by laypersons affected by disabilities, who were organized by the Hastings Center, a bioethics think tank.[16] The disability community's critique of prenatal testing asserts (1) that prenatal genetic testing followed by selective abortion is morally problematic and (2) that the choice of prenatal genetic testing followed by abortion is driven by misinformation. Although a consensus on all issues raised by the disability community was not reached, an endorsement was given to the recommendation to reform how prenatal genetic testing information is communicated to prospective parents. Rather than have prenatal genetic test information and consent as part of the routine first postconception visit and become somewhat trivialized, the recommendation is to provide more time, with the intent of making prenatal genetic testing more thoughtful and considered. For example, if prenatal genetic testing is discussed in the same visit and with the same emphasis as gestational diabetes testing, the parents may not understand all the ramifications of prenatal genetic testing. The disability community also recommended that when parents face the birth of a child with a potential disability, they be given information of what life is like with such a child and not have the spoken or unspoken medical recommendation be termination of the pregnancy.

The role of nurses in obtaining informed consent before a prenatal genetic test is to have a critical time of interaction with the prospective parents. This discussion must include the benefits and risks for the parents and the offspring, the decisions that will be present in the face of a genetic test that indicates risk of disease/disability, the potential for a result that leaves uncertainty to the degree of risk for the offspring, and the recognition that connecting genetic test results (genotype) indicating potential disease with actual symptoms (phenotype) of the disease is not yet possible in most cases. Whether the prospective parents accept or decline prenatal genetic testing and/or termination, it is important that nurses put aside their personal values in the face of such difficult decisions and provide accurate and sensitive information to their patients.

### Diagnostic Genetic Testing

Diagnostic genetic testing is typically done after symptoms of a given disease have been found. If a disease has a genetic basis, the implication is that the family is at risk. Nurses have always been aware that although an individual may be affected by the condition, families are the unit of care. Such awareness is critical when genomics is part of the individual's condition. Research on young women who carry a genetic mutation for hereditary breast and ovarian cancer illustrates the importance of understanding how the family is affected by genetic risk.[17,18] This quote from a 28-year-old woman illustrates how a diagnosis of breast cancer and a genetic test showing a mutation in the BRCA1 gene affects not only her but also her sisters and her parents:

> I have three sisters (age 21, 23, 27) they now have to worry about genetic counseling and possible testing and mammograms. I feel guilty (strangely enough) because I am the one that brought this out in the open. While not said out loud, I think it weighs heavy on my parents because "it came from them." My family is no longer as lighthearted as we once were. Genetic discussions happen all the time. I feel like there is absolutely no escaping this disease. And I know that the chances of having to watch someone I love go through this are high and that breaks my heart.

Nurses who interact with young women who test positive for the BRCA1 or BRCA2 mutation need to appreciate that although a diagnosis of breast cancer at a young age is in itself very difficult, having a genetic mutation specific to the disease amplifies the impact and concerns well beyond that individual.

### Presymptomatic Genetic Testing

Presymptomatic genetic testing occurs before the onset of a disease but within a family that has a history of a given disease.[12] For example, an individual whose parent has Huntington disease (HD) may want to know if they too carry the gene mutation. HD is an autosomal dominant neurodegenerative disorder resulting in irreversible progressive loss of cognitive, motor, and behavioral functioning that lasts 10 to 25 years after the symptoms begin. Signs of the condition most commonly appear between the ages of 30 and 50 years, and individuals with HD lose their abilities to carry out responsibilities as wage earners, spouses, parents, and eventually the ability to care for themselves.[19] Although professionals may think that individuals at risk for HD want to know their risk status, only 5% to 20% of individuals at risk for HD have been tested.[20] Nurses need to be sensitive as to why their patients at risk for an adult-onset genetic disease may not wish to be tested. In the case of HD, there is no effective treatment, individuals cannot "undo" the knowledge that they will develop this devastating disease, that they have potential insurance discrimination, and that reproductive choices may be made more difficult.[21] Also individuals may disrupt their own families by finding out that they do not carry the HD mutation although their siblings are still at risk (Hamilton RJ. Experiencing predictive genetic testing in families with Huntington's disease and hereditary breast and ovarian cancer [Dissertation]. Madison (WI): Unpublished dissertation; 2003).[22] Participants in a study talked about the losses they experienced after finding out they do not have the mutation for HD:

*I also feel a sense of loss in my own family. Things changed that day (she received a negative HD test result), and I was not prepared for the loneliness that I would feel. I don't feel like the same sister that shared the fear about our futures (siblings). Now being happy for my own future seems selfish and fearing for their future seems condescending. Even with my sister that I am very close to, we no longer speak of Huntington's. We use to joke around about sharing a nursing home room and now I know she keeps her feelings to herself. And I feel that any attempts to empathize will not be interpreted in the same way they use to.*

Once again it is critical that nurses understand the larger implications of genetic testing. Research has shown that although most patients are appreciative of knowing that they carry a mutation that increases their risk for a particular disease, they also speak of a "before" and "after." They describe their lives and that of their families as different after genetic testing, and an appreciation of such an impact is critical for nurses who engage patients anywhere along the trajectory of a genetic diagnosis.[17,18] Understanding the potential ripple effects that surround genetic testing in families is important. It may be the case that only 1 person in the family has the genetic test, but by doing so, the implications of an inheritable genetic disease is brought to the foreground.[23] Genetic disease is a family affair, and nurses must be prepared to engage not only the individual patient but also other family members.

Issues of family changes after genetic testing, including fears of future disease and disease in siblings and offspring are inherent. Difficulty living with the knowledge of risk for a potential future disease onset, fears of discrimination and stigmatization, and wondering if the hope for genetic-based therapies is realistic are just a few examples of the worries manifested by patients. Nurses who have a sound knowledge base in the science and who understand the implications of genetic information are better prepared to provide high-quality care in this new area.

**WHEN TO ACT**

Nursing is a practice discipline, and so it is by actions that nurses manifest their professionalism. To act in this postgenomic age requires an awareness and appreciation for the complexities and uniqueness of genetic information. As understanding of gene-gene and gene-environment interaction increases, the complexities of disease prevention, diagnosis, and prognosis will increase. Recognizing this, nurses must act with the greatest sensitivity and discretion in managing genetic information. Although issues of privacy and confidentiality are always important in health care, it is difficult to overstate their importance relative to genetic information of a patient. The role of the nurse in obtaining informed consent for any procedure that requires the collection and analyzing of an individual's DNA goes hand-in-hand with actions protecting the privacy and confidentiality of patient information. Patients must understand what type of information they will receive, who will have access to this information, what happens to their DNA after the test is done, and how the test results will benefit and/or potentially harm them and their family.

In 2006, a consensus panel cochaired by Jean Jenkins of the NHGRI and Kathleen Calzone of the NCI published a set of essential genetic competencies that apply to all RNs.[2] These competencies reflect the minimal knowledge set expected of an RN. At the time of their publication, these competencies were endorsed by multiple nursing organizations, including the ANA and the ANCC, and 2 colleges of nursing. Examples of actions that nurses can take and the corresponding competency (shown in quotes) in relation to genetic information about their patients include:

- Manage genetic information
  - o "Advocate for the rights of all clients for autonomous, informed genetic and genomic-related decision making and voluntary action"
- Refer a patient to genetics specialists when appropriate
  - o "Facilitates referrals for specialized genetic and genomic services for clients as needed"
- Educate patients about genetics
  - o "Provides clients with credible, accurate, appropriate, and current genetic and genomic information, resources, services, and/or technologies that facilitate decision making"
- Work for equal access for all patients to genetic services
  - o "Advocate for clients access to desired genetic/genomic services and/or resources including support groups"

To act as a nurse means to engage in informed practice with knowledge and expertise. In genomic health care, taking action and being aware of the implications of those actions is part of an ethically informed practice. To better understand how the expected competencies may be performed, examples of each action are briefly discussed.

## Manage Genetic Information

An early document[24] published by the ANA addressed the need for nurses to actively protect patients' genetic information. Professional nursing conduct as described in the nursing code of ethics[25] addresses protection of patient information; early in the Human Genome Project process, leaders in nursing, other health care fields, and bioethics[26] recognized that genetic information was in some ways unique. Examples given for the uniqueness of genetic information include (1) genetics yields vast amounts of personal data about an individual, (2) screening and testing can give information about future health risks, (3) screening and testing may yield information about other family members, and (4) DNA samples can be stored and analyzed in the future.[24] The first 2 examples can be illustrated as follows: although a blood test for cholesterol levels will tell an individual whether or not his or her level is normal, a genetic test for an alteration in the *APOE* gene may not only indicate that an individual has an exceptionally high risk for high cholesterol levels and heart disease but also indicate a risk for

Alzheimer disease (AD).[27] An individual who simply wants to know if he or she is at risk for coronary artery disease (CAD) may not welcome information about risk for AD. The type and amount of data available from an individual's genome is unmatched by other medical tests. Nurses who have access to genetic information must be aware of and sensitive to what it is their patient is actually seeking and not overstep by conveying more information or providing more education than what is sought.

The example of *APOE* testing also illustrates that a genetic test may indicate that siblings, offsprings, and other extended family may also be at risk for CAD and AD.[28] The US health care system strongly supports patient autonomy. However, because genetic information is familial in nature, it complicates notions of individuals' autonomy and brings new complexities to the management of health information. Questions have risen regarding whether or not health care providers are responsible for notifying family members of their patients who have tested positive for a gene mutation that significantly increases the risk for disease.[29,30] Research largely indicates that individuals who obtain their genetic test results will disclose this information to selected family members although it may be over a longer period of time than might be expected.[17,31–33] Nurses must realize that genetic information often takes on a quality for the patient and family, above and beyond typical medical information. Being cognizant of the patient's privacy and the confidentiality of the information is central to nursing care in this postgenomic age.

Finally, DNA may be stored and analyzed in the future, which could lead to breeches of privacy and informed consent if such use extends beyond that which was originally provided. The question of who "owns" the DNA sample[34–36] has been raised. A DNA sample may be stored with identifying information or may be deidentified, raising other questions, such as who has access to stored DNA, what tests may be run on the sample in the future, who retains rights of ownership of the samples, and whether there is a duty to the "owner" to be kept informed of future test results. The critical job of the nurse is to be certain that the informed consent process is thorough and provides understandable information to the patient as to the purpose of the genetic test, the risks and benefits, how the results and subsequent information will be handled, what happens to the DNA sample in the future, if there is any secondary use of the genetic material, and if the patient and/or family will have access to future research discoveries in which their DNA was used.[2,24] Nurses are often responsible for ensuring the adequacy of the informed consent procedures, and it is critical that they understand the larger picture of genetic information to adequately advocate for their patients in this area.

### Refer a Patient to Genetics Specialists when Appropriate

One of the professional practices specifically addressed in the *Essential Nursing Competencies for Genetics and Genomics*[2] is for the RN to "facilitate referrals for specialized genetic and genomic services for clients as needed". This action requires 2 elements: (1) recognizing when the patient has a potential genetic condition and (2) recognizing that the setting in which the nurse is seeing the patient is not sufficient to address the genetic concerns of that patient. Examples of an infection-control RN and a family nurse practitioner (FNP) in a retail health clinic illustrate this particular action. The first example shows the incorporation of pharmacogenetics, which is the study of drug reactions based on genetic makeup. The second example indicates the renewed interest and acknowledgment of the importance of a 3-generation family history assessment in primary care settings.

An infection-control RN, Ruth, is working in a community health clinic that manages the weekly medication administration of isoniazid for tuberculosis patients. One of

Ruth's patients has been consistently complaining of numbness in his hands and feet. The dosage of isoniazid has been checked and is appropriate for the weight of this patient. Because Ruth has completed some continuing education units on pharmaco-genetics and knows that drug metabolism is directed by genes, she begins to suspect that her patient may be a "slow acetylator" of isoniazid caused by a mutation in the genes that code for the enzyme *N*-acetyltransferase. Ruth recommends that her patient's acetylator status be determined and in the meantime administers pyridoxine because this drug prevents the peripheral neuropathy secondary to high serum levels of isoniazid.[37,38]

Jeff is an FNP in a retail health clinic in a branch of a nationwide drug store. Recently, the company has required, as part of the intake assessment, a 3-generation family history for cardiac diseases, cancers, and diabetes. Jeff's first patient of the day is a 25-year-old woman, in for a complaint of a sore throat. However, while doing the family history, it is evident that this patient's family has several occurrences of breast cancer with an onset before the age of 50 years. The patient tells Jeff that she is aware of this but does not really know what to do and has not ever had a consistent primary care doctor. Because Jeff knows that certain gene mutations (*BRCA1* and *BRCA2*) are associated with early-onset breast cancer and ovarian cancer and that this patient's family history indicates that she may be at risk for having such mutations, he gives her information about local genetic counseling services and recommends that she follows up with a genetic counselor to have her risk evaluated.

As more genetic tests and pharmacogenetic information becomes available, nurses will have to assess what they know and when it is appropriate to refer their patients to genetic specialists.

### Educate Patients About Genetics

Except for a few well-elucidated mutations, little is actually known about what genes with any certainty predict disease. For example, although several genes have been associated with the development of type 2 diabetes, none of them are predictive to any degree.[39] Time magazine's number one invention of the year in 2008[40] was the company 23andMe, who for $399 will sequence an individual's genome and provide a picture of disease risk, ancestry, and traits (https://www.23andme.com/). Such direct-to-consumer testing opens a host of concerns for health care providers.[41] Although such information may be interesting and exciting to the layperson, nurses have the added responsibility of being able to help patients interpret what such infor-mation means. The proliferation of genetic information that can now be purchased "over the counter" is interesting but largely unspecific and, for that reason, not much help at present in predicting future health.[41] Science has not advanced to the point of predicting future health, and for nurses to be able to educate their patients about what a genetic test result actually means, they must be aware of the difference between commercial science information (such as 23andMe and others) and actual substantiated research results.[42] If the Human Genome Project lives up to the health care community's expectations, individual genomes will provide information about risk for disease, health resiliency, personal pharmacogenetics, potential gene therapy for diagnosed diseases, and other information.[43]

### Work for Equal Access for all Patients to Genetic Services

In a policy statement, ISONG addresses the question of equal access to genetic services: "Nurses share with other health care professionals the responsibility to ensure equal access to genetic information and genomic health care services."[44] Applying the Code of Ethics for nurses by the ICN[45] and the ANA,[25] this position statement points out nurses' responsibility to initiate and promote efforts to ensure the health of the public. As genetic advances continue in disease prediction, diagnoses, and treatment, it is essential that all individuals in need of such services have access to them. In the United States, those with little or no health insurance may have limited opportunity to access genetic health services. ISONG recommends several actions in which nurses can engage to work toward equal access for genetic services, some of which are:

- Recognize and acknowledge the role of genomics as an integral component in the promotion of the public's health and well-being.
- Advocate and promote the right of the individual or family to voluntarily choose or not choose to seek genomic health care services.
- Evaluate and support legislation that provides protection from health insurance and employment discrimination at the state and federal levels.
- Identify and seek solutions to the elimination of barriers to accessing genetic health care.
- Advocate equal access to genomic health care.[44]

Well-informed nurses can significantly affect the public discussion of access to genetic services.

One barrier to the access of genetic health services in the United States was removed when President Bush signed the Genetic Information Nondiscrimination Act (GINA) on May 21, 2008.[46] After a 13-year battle in Congress, this federal law protects Americans against discrimination based on their genetic information when it comes to health insurance and employment. The New York Times reported in February 2008[47] that individuals who already had symptoms of a disease and those who felt they had a significant risk for a genetic disease were deciding against genetic testing because of fears of insurance discrimination. GINA potentiates the possibility for people to take full advantage of the promise of personalized medicine without fear of discrimination.

## SUMMARY

Nurses have entered the postgenomic age as professionals expected to engage with the public and provide informed up-to-date genetic information and competencies. Along with their colleagues, they will need to continue to educate themselves in the area of genomics as they respond to the needs of their patients and families. Nursing is a practice discipline, and so it is by actions that nurses manifest their profession-alism. To act in this postgenomic age requires an awareness and appreciation for the complexities and uniqueness of genetic information.

As the understanding of gene-gene and gene-environment interaction increases, the complexities of disease prevention, diagnosis, and prognosis will increase. Recognizing this, nurses must act with the greatest sensitivity and discretion in managing genetic information. Although issues of privacy and confidentiality are always important in health care, it is difficult to overstate their importance relative to genetic information of a patient. The role of the nurse in obtaining informed consent for any procedure that requires the collection and analyzing of an individual's DNA goes hand-in-hand with actions protecting the privacy and confidentiality of patient information. Patients must understand what type of information they will receive, who will have access to this information, what happens to their DNA after the test is done, and how the test results will benefit and/or potentially harm them and their family.

Finally, the promises of genomic health care will only be realized if everyone has access to the technologies and improved outcomes. Equal access to health care is a challenge in the United States. Equal access to genetic-based health care is no less so and has barriers beyond that of other health care services. Nurses have an obligation to work to remove such barriers so that all individuals who could benefit from genomic health care have the opportunity to do so.

Genomics will drive the health care advances throughout the twenty-first century. As the largest health care provider group and the provider group that interacts most closely with the patient, nurses have an obligation to be knowledgeable, to reason critically, and to act with skill and sensitivity in the area of genomics. It is an exciting challenge and an opportunity for nurses and their patients.

## ACKNOWLEDGMENTS

I would like to thank my colleagues at the University of Illinois at Chicago, College of Nursing, Drs. Agatha Gallo and Patricia Herschberger for their careful reading and helpful suggestions on the early drafts of this article.

## REFERENCES

1. Collins FS. The human genome project and the future of medicine. Ann N Y Acad Sci 1999;882:42–55.
2. Consensus Panel on Genetic/Genomic Nursing Competencies. Essential nursing competencies and curricula guidelines for genetics and genomics. Silver Spring (MD): American Nurses Association; 2006.
3. United States Department of Health and Human Services. (2004). The Registered Nurse Population: Findings from the 2004 National Sample Survey of Registered Nurses. Available at: http://bhpr.hrsa.gov/healthworkforce/rnsurvey04/. Accessed November 21, 2008.
4. NHGRI. Human Genome Project. Available at: http://www.genome.gov/10001772. Accessed November 20, 2008, 2008.
5. Anderson G, Monsen RB, Prows CA, et al. Preparing the nursing profession for participation in a genetic paradigm in health care. Nurs Outlook 2000;48(1): 23–7.
6. ISONG. Mission statement. Available at: http://www.isong.org/about/index.cfm. Accessed November 21, 2008.
7. Scanlon C, Fibison W. Managing genetic information: implication for nursing practice. Washington, DC: American Nurses Publishing; 1995.
8. NCHPEG. Core competencies in genetics essential for all health care professionals. Available at: http://www.nchpeg.org/core. Accessed June 26, 2002.
9. Jenkins J, Calzone K. Establishing the essential nursing competencies for genetics and genomics. J Nurs Scholarsh 2007;39(1):10–6.
10. American Association of Colleges of Nursing. The essentials of Baccalaureate education for professional nursing practice. Washington, DC: American Association of Colleges of Nursing; 2008.
11. Feetham SL, Williams JK, editors. Genetics in nursing. 1st edition. Geneva, Switzerland: International Council of Nurses; 2004.
12. Guttmacher AE, Collins FS. Genomic medicine – a primer. N Engl J Med 2002; 347(19):1512–20.
13. Lashley FR. Genetics in nursing education. Nurs Clin North Am 2000;35(3): 795–805.

14. Thomson EJ. Ethical, legal, social, and policy issues in genetics. In: Lashley FR, editor. The genetics revolution: implications for nursing. Washington, DC: American Academy of Nursing; 1997. p. 15–26.
15. ELSI. A review and analysis of the ethical, legal, and social implications research programs at the National Institutes of Health and Department of Energy: final report of the ELSI Research Planning and Evaluation Group [Online]. Available at: http://www.doe.gov. Accessed February 10, 2000.
16. Parens E, Asch A, editors. Prenatal testing and disability rights. 1st edition. Washington, DC: Georgetown University Press; 2000.
17. Hamilton RJ, Bowers BJ, Williams JK. Disclosing genetic test results to family members. J Nurs Scholarsh 2005;37(1):18–24.
18. Hamilton RJ, Williams JK, Bowers BJ, et al. Life trajectories, genetic testing, and risk reduction decisions in 18–39 year old women at risk for hereditary breast and ovarian cancer. J Genet Couns 2009;18:147–59.
19. Rosenblatt A, Ranen NG, Nance MA, et al. A physician's guide to the management of Huntington's disease. 2nd edition. New York: Huntington's Disease Society of America; 1999.
20. Oster E, Dorsey ER, Bausch J, et al. Fear of health insurance loss among individuals at risk for Huntington disease. Am J Med Genet 2008;146A:2070–7.
21. Quaid KA, Morris M. Reluctance to undergo predictive testing: the case of Huntington disease. Am J Med Genet 1993;45:41–5.
22. Williams JK, Schutte DL, Evers C, et al. Redefinition: coping with normal results from predictive gene testing for neurodegenerative disorders. Res Nurs Health 2000;23:260–9.
23. Hamilton RJ, Bowers BJ. The theory of genetic vulnerability: a Roy model exemplar. Nurs Sci Q 2007;20(3):254–65.
24. Scanlon C, Fibison W. Managing genetic information: implications for nursing practice. Washington, DC: American Nurses Publishing; 1995.
25. American Nurses Association. Code for nurses with interpretive statements. Washington, DC: American Nurses Association; 1985.
26. Collins F. Shattuck lecture-medical and societal consequences of the human genome project. N Engl J Med 1999;341(1):28–37.
27. Bertram L, Tanzi RE. The genetic epidemiology of neurodegenerative disease. J Clin Invest 2005;115(6):1449–57.
28. Quaid KA. Implications of genetic susceptibility testing with Apolipoprotien E. In: Post SG, Whitehouse PJ, editors. Genetic testing for Alzheimer disease: ethical and clinical issues. Baltimore (MD): John Hopkins University Press; 1998. p. 118–39.
29. Dugan RB, Weisner GL, Juengst ET, et al. Duty to warn at-risk relatives for genetic disease: genetic counselors' clinical experience. Am J Med Genet C Semin Med Genet 2003;119C:27–34.
30. Hallowell N, Foster C, Eeles R, et al. Balancing autonomy and responsibility: the ethics of generating and disclosing genetic information. J Med Ethics 2003;29(2): 74–91.
31. Hallowell N, Ardern-Jones A, Eeles R, et al. Communication about genetic testing in families of male BRCA1/2 carriers and non-carriers: patterns, priorities and problems. Clin Genet 2005;67:492–502.
32. Forrest K, Simpson SA, Wilson BJ, et al. To tell or not to tell: barriers and facilitators in family communication about genetic risk. Clin Genet 2003;64:317–26.
33. Wilson BJ, Forrest K, van Teijlingen ER, et al. Family communication about genetic risk: the little that is known. Community Genet 2004;7:15–24.

34. Roche PA. Caveat venditor: protecting privacy and ownership interests in DNA. In: Knoppers BM, editor. Human DNA: law & policy. Springer; 1997. p. 33–41.

35. Annas GJ, Glantz LH, Roche PA. Drafting the Genetic Privacy Act: science, policy, and practical considerations. J Law Med Ethics 1995;23:360–6.

36. Williams S. "Who owns your genes?" event illuminates arguments for and against DNA patenting. Biotech Briefing 2007;4:3–6.

37. Prows CA, Prows DR. Medication selection by genotype: How genetics is changing drug prescribing and efficacy. Am J Nurs 2004;104(8):16.

38. Lashley FR. Clinical genetics in nursing practice. 3rd edition. New York: Springer Publishing Company; 2005.

39. Florez JC. The genetics of type 2 diabetes: a realistic appraisal CIRCA 2008. Journal of Clinical Endocrine Metabolism 2008;93:4633–42.

40. Hamilton A. Time's best inventions of 2008. Time 2008;10:68–9.

41. Hudson K, Javitt G, Burke W, et al. ASHG statement on direct-to-consumer genetic testing in the United States. Am J Hum Genet 2007;81:635–7.

42. Prows CA. Clinical aspects of genomics: an update. Online J Issues Nurs 2008; 131(1). Available at: www.nursingworld.org/MainMenuCategories/ANAMarket-place/ANAPeriodicals/OJIN/TableofContents/vol132008/No1Jan08/ClinicalAspects ofGenomics.aspx. Accessed October 14, 2009.

43. Collins FS, Green ED, Guttmacher AE, et al. A vision for the future of genomics research. Nature 2003;422:835–47.

44. ISONG. Position statement: access to genomic healthcare: the role of the nurse. Available at: http://www.isong.org/about/ps_genomic.cfm. 2003. Accessed November 20, 2008.

45. International Council of Nurses. The ICN code of ethics for nurses. Geneva, Switzerland: ICN; 2000.

46. NHGRI. Genetic Non-Discrimination Act. Available at: http://www.genome.gov/24519851. Accessed November 20, 2008.

47. Harmon A. THE DNA AGE; fear of insurance trouble leads many to shun or hide DNA tests. New York Times February 24, 2008.

# Healing During Existential Moments: The "Art" of Nursing Presence

Karen Iseminger, PhD, FNP[a],*, Francesca Levitt, MSN, RN-BC, CNS[b],
Lisa Kirk, RN, BSN, CWOCN[c]

**KEYWORDS**

- Nursing presence • Transformative nursing presence model
- Caring • Connectedness • Nurse-patient relationship
- Spiritual formation

The essence of clinical nursing practice is to provide comfort and healing by attending to patients' physical, emotional, and spiritual needs. This involves balancing the art of nursing with the science of nursing. During the last half century, scholars have championed the science component of the art/science duo. At times, undervaluing emotional and spiritual care may occur because of time limitations or fear of vulnerability. The elevation of the art of nursing presence to equal status in the profession empowers the nurse to unite empiric ways of knowing with existential ways of being. Actualizing the concept of nursing presence allows nurses to use empiric and metaphysical knowledge about better ways to meet holistic needs of patients. Nursing presence is foundational to the establishment of therapeutic relationships and is instrumental in improving personal and professional satisfaction.

## NURSING PRESENCE, HEALING, EXISTENTIALISM, AND THE ART OF NURSING

In a review of the literature on nursing presence, Doona and colleagues[1] noted inconsistency in the use of the term "nursing presence." Drawing on concepts in existential philosophy, they proposed defining nursing presence as "an intersubjective encounter between a nurse and a patient in which the nurse encounters the patient as a unique human being in a unique situation and chooses to spend herself on his behalf. ... an intense intersubjective reality that permanently changes the participants."[2] This

[a] St. Vincent Health, 10330 North Meridian Street, Suite 380, Indianapolis, IN 46290-1024, USA
[b] St. Vincent Hospital, 2001 West 86th Street, Indianapolis, IN 46260, USA
[c] Clarian Health Partners, Riley Hospital for Children, 702 Barnhill Drive, ROC Rm 2208, Indianapolis, IN 46202, USA
* Corresponding author.
*E-mail address:* kaisemin@stvincent.org (K. Iseminger).

Nurs Clin N Am 44 (2009) 447–459
doi:10.1016/j.cnur.2009.07.001
0029-6465/09/$ – see front matter © 2009 Elsevier Inc. All rights reserved.

nursing.theclinics.com

definition includes spatial and temporal aspects, where the nurse faces the patient and holds out the gift of a caring interaction. Nursing presence includes empathy, caring, holistic care, and attentiveness, but these terms are inadequate to fully capture the essence of nursing presence. Nursing presence represents more than an expression connoting an aspiration for something beyond objective analyses of the current situation.[3] Nursing scholars, such as Ellen Olshansky, appreciate that an orientation to awe, recognition of a divine presence, or acknowledgment of mystery may be manifest even during mundane events and is vital to the art of nursing.[4]

The term the art of nursing (presence) as discussed by Finfgeld-Connett[5] describes the "expert use and adaptation of empiric and metaphysical knowledge and values." It is contrasted with the science of nursing, which consists of empiric knowledge resulting from established research methodologies. Metaphysical knowledge refers to "less formally acquired insights which depend on our unconscious ability to process information - extract data from various sources, preprocess it and act on the results. This form of knowledge includes an astute awareness of things that are not always visible, audible, or palpable."[5] Thus, the artful nurse is one who augments traditional nursing processes with an awareness of the appreciation of mystery.* "Being with," an essential nursing orientation, entails extensive knowledge of the patient and being responsive to the unique patient at an exact moment in time. According to Patterson and Zderad,[6] being with requires turning attention toward the patient, being aware of and open to the here and now and the shared situation, while communicating availability to another in the form of being present.

Prerequisites to establishing presence are self-awareness, openness, flexibility, and a willingness to embrace another's situation—the same factors that Anne Williams includes in quality nursing care.[7] Williams describes "selective focusing" as occurring when the nurse attempts to balance self-awareness and therapeutically effective nursing care with time demands. Care and empathy enable caregivers to recognize suffering or need without losing themselves in the other person.[8] Self-reflection allows the nurse to maintain a sense of self and a clear distinction between caregiver and patient. An empathic relationship fosters collaboration, cooperation, and healing, whereas one that reduces the patient to that of an object may add additional emotional injury to the patients' suffering.

> *A quadriplegic patient was admitted to treat a pressure ulcer. While doing the initial assessment, the nurse commented, "It doesn't look that bad." The patient advised the nurse that while his might not be the worst pressure ulcer ever, this one had devastating effects on the patient's daily life, independence, and ability to work. Had the nurse been 'present' to this patient, she would have empathized with the person instead of simply treating the wound, thus effecting better emotional and physical healing. (Lisa Kirk, RN, BSN, Indianapolis, IN, personal experience, 2008)*

According to Finfgeld-Connett,[9] nursing presence requires the recipient's openness and need for presence and the nurse's willingness to share. Women in labor commonly described nurses' presence as being there (physically present), being with (going beyond, acknowledging a mystery also present), and being for them (advocacy).[10] Lennart Fredriksson offers a compelling picture of the difference between "being with" (a deeper and more vulnerable gift of self in the encounter) versus "being there" (a physical presence that encompasses communication and understanding).[11]

---

* Our usage of mystery implies a belief in something 'more than' objective reality—'beyond human understanding'—and is made known by divine revelation. It also refers to 'God' or 'Higher Power.'

Presence and caring is a therapeutic process that includes expert nursing practice (assessment, decision making, and intervention) in addition to intimate interpersonal sensitivity. This sensitivity is demonstrated by eye contact, appropriate touching, and focusing on patient needs. The benefits to recipients of caring and presence are an improvement in mental and physical well-being. Personal and professional maturity are requisite to nursing presence; they include a commitment to help in a respectful, nonjudgmental manner, regardless of circumstances.

Edward Farley[12] says empathy is a transcendent phenomenon that involves being with others. Some nurses perceive this type of interaction to be less important and more difficult than traditional nursing tasks. Nevertheless, the act of being with and the administration of competent traditional physical care tasks are crucial to being an effective nurse and instrumental in creating a healing presence. Healing is defined as the integration of psychological, physical, spiritual, and social components, which are beneficial even when a cure is impossible.[13] A therapeutic relationship is a partnership between the nurse and patient involving personal qualities and caregiving skills, skilled communication, respect for autonomy and diversity, and shared decision making.[14] Effective nurse-patient interaction is easier for some nurses than others because of different personalities, education, beliefs, self-awareness, and communication styles. The challenges associated with creating meaningful relationships with patients and families require effort, energy, and moral courage.

To elaborate on this concept, we draw on the work of the French phenomenologist, Emmanuel Levinas.[15] Levinas holds that intersubjectivity is necessary but insufficient to describe the appropriate stance between the *Self* (the nurse) and the *Other* (the patient). Levinas portrays the complexity of the *Other* through the face, or visage. For him, the face of the *Other* is a unique locus of expressivity. Through experiencing the face of the *Other*, the world is opened up and made manifest to others. In face-to-face encounters, the face of the *Other* is a source of meanings and the epiphany of infinite transcendence, expressed as a holy language. Levinas's notion of *vers l'etranger* (toward the foreigner) is his symbolic representation that truth comes from the outside from afar and abroad; that the "foreigner" or mystery within us helps us to experience truth in relationship to others. Intersubjectivity offers the subject and the object of perception, a method by which to discern the similarities and disparities between their consciousnesses. On this point, Adrian Van Kaam[16] holds that when we fully attend to others, we can be involved in everyday activities while at the same time transcending them.

Focusing on the existential *Other* demonstrates a desire to elevate the nurse-patient relationship from an impersonal provider studying the object to one that does not reduce patients to object status but transforms the relationship into a dynamic partnership. Moreover, Levinas advocates a turn to transcendence, welcoming the patient (*Other*), requiring nurses to forego egoistic stances. The following passage from Jill Bolte Taylor describing her experience as a stroke patient beautifully demonstrates not only this welcoming practice but also the reciprocal power of the nurse's visage:

*With this shift into my right hemisphere, I became empathic to what others felt. Although I could not understand the words they spoke, I could read volumes from their facial expression and body language. I paid very close attention to how energy dynamics affected me. I realized that some people brought me energy while others took it away. One nurse was very attentive to my needs ... naturally, I felt very safe in her care. She made eye contact and was clearly providing me with a healing space. A different nurse, who never made eye contact, shuffled her feet as though she were in pain. ... Under the circumstances, her lack of willingness to connect with me scared me. I did not feel safe in her care.*[17]

## PERCEIVED BARRIERS TO ACTUALIZING NURSING PRESENCE

Barriers to actualizing nursing presence are associated with perceived time constraints related to low staffing ratios, high patient acuity, discomfort with intense, meaningful communication, and perceived low value of the activity. However, when nurses are truly present to patients, they can act proactively, clustering care and increasing efficiency, thereby reducing patients' additional calls for assistance. Perhaps the patients' perception of nursing presence can be achieved in seconds rather than minutes. By including patients as partners in their care, their anxiety may be reduced, and a better healing environment fostered.

Nurses' peers may also discourage nursing presence. When others observe their colleagues spending too much time with patients, they may think that the nurse is struggling with time management, when in fact they are consciously and purposely spending time interacting and being with patients. Thus, it is not uncommon for nurses to change units or hospitals to find a supportive, like-minded environment that reinforces the value of nursing presence. A study on the correlation between an ethical climate and job satisfaction of nurses, reported by Ulrich and colleagues,[18] substantiates this claim. They discovered that most of their respondents reported that respect in the workplace and a belief in the institutional mission are more important factors for nurse retention than salary and staffing.

When faced with economic challenges, individuals may enter the nursing profession merely as a means to financial security rather than a desire to help others. Thus, another barrier to nursing presence arises when the desire to connect is absent (impoverished motivation) or has been eroded. Erosion equates with attitudes such as indifference, apathy, going through the motions, and disengagement. Furthermore, the disconnected nurse may contend, "nursing is just a job," "I need the money and benefits," or "It doesn't make any difference anyway." The Van Kaam[16] and Muto[19] response to this erosion involves strategies that foster dispositional change (empathic appreciation, respectful listening, and joy, ie, the sense of awe, in the midst of the situation). Moreover, some nurses create professional distance to protect themselves from experiencing patients' suffering or facing their own vulnerability and mortality.

## CARING, NURSING PRESENCE, AND SPIRITUALITY

Nursing literature on caring and nursing presence is often associated with spirituality. A review of the literature in the categories of conceptual and theory development, clinical application, and nursing education revealed that the concepts of nurses caring for themselves, patient advocacy, and moral agency are interrelated. Some believe that evolving holistic nursing requires teaching spirituality and nursing presence in nursing programs. Others argue that presence is a developmental skill, first identified in practice and then evolving as the nurse matures professionally.[20]

To increase awareness of interactions that exemplify nursing presence and to develop intuitive awareness, faculty at a mid-Atlantic university provided nursing students with instructor-guided reflections after each clinical experience. The reflection activities encouraged students to explore and further develop an understanding of themselves as spiritual beings and to examine concepts of spiritual care and nursing presence in light of their clinical experience. These exercises allowed students to integrate their learning experience into a comprehensive perception (self-discovery) of their role as spiritual caregivers.[20]

In a qualitative study at the School of Nursing at the University of Athens, Greece, students kept a journal of their clinical experiences. Themes of the encounters included empathizing with patients and empathizing and identifying with nurses. Other themes included disillusionment with nursing practice when encountering ethical misconduct. This fostered moral awakening and the development of moral and professional personhood. Still other themes described transcending the conventional ethics of the unit and attaining moral satisfaction through actualization of good practice. The authors recommended providing students with opportunities to reflect and with psychological and peer support. Additional interventions included role modeling, storytelling, journaling, and interviewing during clinical experiences.[21]

Presence, of which spirituality is a significant component, is described as caring, holistic care, therapeutic relationship, trust, and communication. Its features include uniqueness, connectedness, sensing, going beyond scientific data, and being with the patient.

## FORMATIVE SPIRITUALITY IN NURSING

Adrian Van Kaam created a spiritual formation model based on the difference between information given and formation achieved. The following observation demonstrates this distinction: "Students take our required ethics courses and pass our tests but no one's behavior changes as a result. ... Introspection, not merely knowledge, is requisite for the formation of a clinician's moral agency, minimizing any disconnection between knowledge and action."[22] Educational systems emphasize imparting information, and thus it is easy to overlook the formative aspects of life-long learning. Formative spirituality is a discipline that provides a way of seeing self and others, life, and world, in light of which we recognize a higher power that is present to us. Van Kaam and Muto describe a transcendence dynamic, the source of which is a formation mystery that does not require someone to be a religious believer. This transcendent process uses appreciative abandonment, a keen sensitivity to what is noticeable in any situation by forsaking total reliance upon oneself in favor of being open to the mystery inherent in "everydayness."[23] If a nurse chooses to use the transcendent practice of appreciative abandonment, then, over time, that would assist in developing the *trait* of presentness (ontologic changes in the nurse-as-moral agent) versus the *state* of presentness (an action of the nurse).[24] Excerpts from an interview with Susan Muto:

> We felt that there was a complete compatibility between many of the constructs and concepts in formation science and formation anthropology that could be invaluable in a curriculum that would attempt to integrate nursing with this more holistic teaching. ... In other words, nurses are desperately searching for meaning, which is what spiritual people do. Even to use one minute of the three minutes you spend with a patient and devote that sixty seconds to something as simple, conveying, 'I am a fellow human being, I have empathy for what you are going through.' (S. Muto, PhD, Pittsburgh, PA, personal communication, 13 November, 2008)

## NURSING PRESENCE AND TRANSCENDENT PRACTICES

Before nurses can make behavior changes reflective of nursing presence, they must first embrace the concept, admit its existence, and acknowledge its importance. Moreover, some nurses may choose transformation via reflective practices, which stimulates the development of character traits that are more conducive to presence. Nurses need to understand that they are instruments of healing and that giving of themselves creates healing in the nurse and the patient. Nurses need to hear that they make a difference, and they need to be commended for their presence, which is as valuable as efficiency and critical-thinking skills.

One way for nurses to achieve enhanced nursing presence is to acknowledge and embrace practices that have been identified as beneficial to good nursing practice in general. The Nursing Interventions Classification (NIC) includes interventions related to nursing presence, such as active listening, anticipatory guidance, anxiety reduction, decision-making support, humor, presence (defined as being with another, physically and psychologically, during times of need), self-efficacy enhancement, and touch.[25] Nurses sharing their authentic selves with patients and families validate their initial decision to choose nursing as a way of helping. Nursing presence demonstrates that a caring attitude can be translated into tangible, meaningful activity. Nurse-sensitive outcomes, such as skin integrity, mobility, and fall prevention, are measures regularly integrated into the daily care of patients. Therapeutic skills associated with nursing presence merit the same recognition as traditional nursing tasks.

Nursing outcomes associated with a therapeutic relationship between patient and nurse, for example, acceptance of health status and client satisfaction, especially as it relates to comfort, hope, and participation in health care decisions, are included in the Nursing Outcomes Classification system (NOC).[26] In addition to the NIC and NOC systems for identifying interventions and outcomes, the Joint Commission now recommend a spiritual assessment.[27] They stipulate that at minimum, the assessment should determine the patient's denomination and significant spiritual beliefs and practices.

Although all nurses have the moral and regulatory responsibility to attend to the spiritual needs of their patients, nurses who choose to work at faith-based organizations may be able to make that connection more overtly. The environment in which the nurse works can be spiritually supportive and uplifting to the entire health care team. Ascension Health, the nation's largest Catholic and largest nonprofit health system in the United States, demonstrates their level of support (**Fig. 1**). This model represents Ascension Health's desire to nurture spirituality in the workplace based on its reverence for each person in the service of his or her healing ministry.

An example of this type of supportive environment can be found at St Vincent Health in Indiana, where many programs and services designed to be enriching and encouraging are available to caregivers.[28] For example, Seton Cove Spirituality Center serves as an ecumenical center for spiritual formation and renewal, with a plethora of classes and retreats that focus on spirituality in the workplace. Healing gardens provide a place of beauty and nature for quiet reflection where staff may reenergize. Accordingly, a therapeutic milieu empowers employees to:

- Find joy in and enjoy their work
- Find meaning and purpose in daily tasks
- Develop a sense of community in their work
- Encourage each other as they serve patients and families
- Deepen their sense of meaning through the mission and values of their ministries.

As individuals find meaning, satisfaction, and a sense of calling, they give faithful, passionate, and excellent service. To merely go through the act of nursing robs the nurse of the abundant gifts that can only come through loving, caring compassion. The goal of fostering a spiritually centered workplace is to help staff connect with the meaning of their work, which encourages individual and organizational transformation from dispassionate care to cohesive holistic care.

The concept of existential advocacy developed by nurse ethicist, Sally Gadow,[29] exemplifies another transcendent practice. It proposes that nurses assist individuals to authentically exercise their freedom of self-determination. Authenticity involves

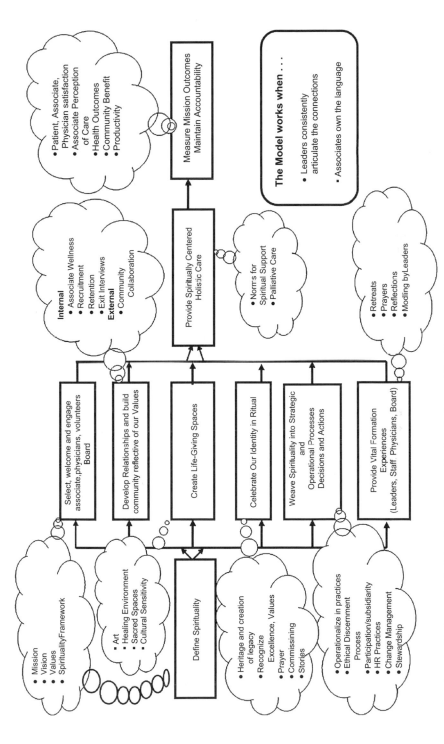

**Fig. 1.** Ascension Health Integral Model, mission integration/workplace spirituality.

reaching decisions that are truly one's own, ones that express all that one believes about oneself and the world, within the entire complexity of one's values. Existential advocacy is an avenue through which the nurse uses metaphysical knowledge (the art of nursing) to cultivate change. As an existential advocate, the nurse must conduct a thorough, holistic assessment of the physical, spiritual, and emotional states of patients and families to create the requisite intersubjectivity needed to appreciate their complex world. An experienced neonatal nurse offers the following application:

> The existential term that has the most significance to me is "becoming." The concept of not only being able to see what one is, but also seeing the possibilities of what one can become. I see on a daily basis families talking of the possibilities for their new baby. They picture their future life; stroller rides, swinging at the park, and the first day of school … long before they ever happen. However, with a significant illness or anomaly [w]e assist the parents to grieve not only for what is, but also for what could have been. (Barbara Hidde, MSN, Indianapolis, IN, personal communication, 2004)

### PROMOTING NURSING PRESENCE: EDUCATIONAL AND CLINICAL APPROACHES

Nursing students and seasoned nurses should always regard patients holistically. The culture of busyness, high patient acuity, and time constraints can compromise holistic practice, making it difficult for nursing students and nurses to value relational skills. If the technical aspects of nursing are overemphasized, nurses' ability to relate to patients is compromised. Finding a balanced synthesis of technical and relational skills is a crucial aspect of nursing education.[30]

Undergraduate nursing educators feel pressured to prepare students for the National Council Licensure Examination (NCLEX) along with teaching technical skills, nursing diagnoses, and care plans. Their focus is on accreditation and basic skills, leaving little time for artful strategies and behaviors. To create meaningful change in the therapeutic milieu, nursing presence should be introduced in the undergraduate classroom and reinforced during nursing orientation, preceptorships, and residency programs, and it should be fully supported and encouraged in mentoring relationships. Special course offerings on the value and benefit of nursing presence should also be available to those interested in personal and professional development.

Graduate nursing education is particularly well suited for additional study of nursing presence because of its increased emphasis on concept analysis and nursing scholarship. Nursing presence in the clinical setting should be established as a critical component of continuing education throughout the nurse's professional life. Advanced practice nurses (APN) can play a significant role in furthering nursing presence in all clinical settings. Nurse practitioners, for example, may serve as a patient's "point of entry" health care provider. As such, they may treat patients for many years; the idea of establishing a therapeutic nursing presence is easily foreseeable. The nurse practitioner's core philosophy is individualized care, which meshes extremely well with the concept of nursing presence. For example, a nurse practitioner–led congestive heart failure clinic used nursing presence to successfully build trust, achieve medical stability, improve compliance, and achieve self-efficacy.[31] Trusting connectedness combined with knowledge of the subjective context of symptoms is a powerful strategy for palliation. Nurses need not fulfill every need expressed by the patient; they must know their limits. However, acknowledging limits should not preclude applying principles of holism.[14]

The clinical nurse specialist (CNS) is in a unique position to support direct caregivers to become more comfortable interacting and communicating with patients. CNSs promote the relationships between nursing presence behaviors and nurse-sensitive outcomes, such as patient satisfaction, nurse satisfaction, and retention. For staff nurses who are interested in professional and personal growth and who are willing to learn about nursing presence, the CNS can observe nursing interactions with patients and role model desirable behaviors conducive to the development of an enhanced therapeutic nurse-patient relationship. The staff nurse can test the water in a nonthreatening real-time environment under the guidance and supervision of the CNS. As a mentor and consultant providing constructive feedback, the CNS may also work to improve the traditional work environment. The CNS works to improve outcomes in 3 spheres of influence: patient, nurse, and organization. By fostering evidence-based practice through sharing the results of quality-improvement projects and published research on the effects of nursing presence, the CNS can demonstrate to staff nurses the connection between nursing presence and patient and organizational benefits.[32]

## Case Study

A certified nurse midwife (CNM), an APN who specializes in obstetrics and gynecology, was present to a woman in premature labor, who was understandably anxious about the unexpected early rupture of membranes:

> The CNM had met the couple seven months ago and had followed the pregnancy throughout the prenatal course. She helped the couple calm down and told them she would meet them at the hospital. After she examined the mother-to-be, who was fully effaced and dilated, the CNM allowed the patient to call her mother in Oklahoma because, at that moment, that personal contact was the most important thing to do. After the phone call, the couple remembers that the whole atmosphere changed dramatically, every muscle relaxed, after three pushes, the baby was born and they all cried tears of joy. During the next two hours, the new parents were left undisturbed with their new baby girl, except for a brief moment when she was bundled to stay warm.
>
> While that phone call to the patient's mother might have seemed like a minor thing, it perfectly exemplifies the quality-of-life approach to health care that recognizes the patient as an existential Other. At that critical moment in the birthing room, this was not simply a 27-year-old primiparous patient, presenting in active labor; she was the Other, whose wishes and longings deserved to be honored.
>
> At other times throughout their pregnancy, the same couple noted a special dimension to the relationship between them and their CNM. Early on, the mother-to-be was anxious while at work. The CNM invited her to come over on her lunch break so she could hear the baby's heartbeat, knowing how reassuring that would be. Amy, the patient stated, "Small gestures, nourished by a relationship that had been cultivated through hours of dialog, earnest listening, and a remarkable openness in attitude transformed a few hours in the hospital into a transcendent experience for my husband and I and our midwife."[33]

## Clinical Practice Examples

Nursing presence in a variety of clinical settings illustrates the benefits realized by patients and their families. In a study of poor pregnant mothers, nursing presence provided an affirming, health-enhancing reciprocal relationship between nurse and client that contributed to the healing of mind, body, and spirit.[34] In conjunction with other interventions, presence is a crucial component of nursing competency. Patients and their families felt more secure when their nurses were present, as manifested by attentiveness, concern, and availability, even in the intensive care unit.[35] In addition to technical skills, nurse managers need to encourage expressive behaviors in their staff.

The ultimate goal is for nurses to become comfortable exhibiting genuine caring, so that they can move from simply providing clinical care, through reflective practices, to having an enhanced presence that fosters healing and positive patient, nurse, and organizational outcomes. This transcendent process is the foundation for the authors' Transformative Nursing Presence (TNP) model (**Fig. 2**), which is described later. Caring nursing behaviors are directly related to patient satisfaction. For example, the nurse caring for oncology patients must be especially present during times when patients' power of self-determination is threatened because a diagnosis of cancer evokes feelings of vulnerability and powerlessness. Characteristic patient responses in these situations include fear, denial, disbelief, despair, distress, anxiety, insomnia, and irritability.[36] The diagnosis frequently provokes patients to reassess their values and life goals.[37] Even when performing seemingly mundane tasks, advocacy nursing dictates participating with patients in determining the personal meaning of their cancer diagnosis and treatment options.

## TOWARD A NEW MODEL: TRANSFORMATIVE NURSING PRESENCE

Most of the literature on nursing presence describes why empathy or presence is crucial and what nursing presence might look like. However, few works address *how* the nurse becomes a person disposed toward being present. Building upon the work of Van Kaam and Muto, which describes the process of spiritual formation (From, Through, To), the authors of this article propose a new approach.[38] Called

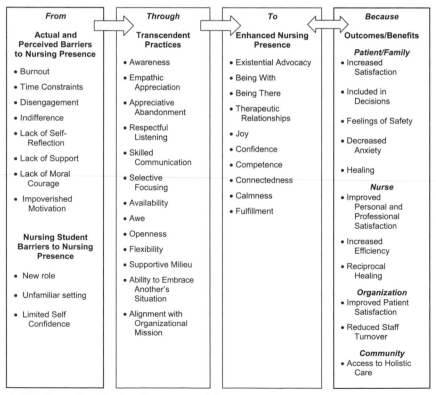

**Fig. 2.** Tranformative Nursing Presence model.

the Transformative Nursing Presence Model and depicted in **Fig. 2**, it includes the following features:

- From: actual and perceived barriers to nursing presence
- Through: transcendent practices
- To: enhanced nursing presence
- Because: the resultant outcomes serve to benefit patients, nurses, organizations, and communities.

The TNP model expands existing scholarship and offers a distinct model to guide nurses and organizations toward establishing enhanced nursing presence. This model illustrates an approach by which a nurse can become present to the patient and offers options to consider as one examines the delivery of exceptional nursing care. This model uses a bidirectional arrow between the "Enhanced Nursing Presence" column and the "Because" column to symbolize the reciprocal relationship that exists between the achievement of outcomes. Thus, nurses benefit by experiencing personal and professional gratification. By creating a culture that supports transcendent nursing practices, organizations may be rewarded with increased nursing retention.

Finally, a significant purpose of any health care organization is to serve the needs of the broader community. Through the provision of holistic care, the community is assured that their individual and collective health care needs will be addressed with sensitivity to body, mind, and spirit. The TNP model is a synthesis of key elements and processes that operationalizes abstract concepts and provides a visual framework to guide nurses and organizations toward outcomes, which benefits patients, nurses, organizations, and the community.

## SUMMARY

This article describes the actual and perceived barriers to nursing presence; these barriers are not insurmountable and should not discourage nurses' desire to find more meaning in their work. Personal transformation from a state of self-centeredness, which leads to eroded social presence, to a state in which one acknowledges greater truth and mystery is possible. Transcendent practices that facilitate nurses' ability to achieve a healing relationship with patients and their families require self-awareness, communication skills, and a supportive work environment.

Enhanced nursing presence results in a greater appreciation of an individuals' subjective experience, through which the patient, the nurse, the organization, and the broader community benefit through the provision of holistic care. Exemplifying the art of nursing presence, the TNP model offers a means for achieving optimal healing during existential moments.

## REFERENCES

1. Doona ME, Chase SK, Haggerty LA. Nursing presence: as real as a milky way bar. J Holist Nurs 1999;17(1):54–70.
2. Doona ME, Haggerty LA, Chase SK. Nursing presence: an existential exploration of the concept. Including commentary by Holzemer, WL. Sch Inq Nurs Pract 1997;11(1):3–20.
3. Louch RK. Formative spiritual glossary of words and phrases from Adrian Van Kaam's Science, anthropology, and theology formation. Pittsburgh (PA): Epiphany Association; 2003. p. 80.

4. Olshansky E. Nursing research in the context of awe and wonder. J Prof Nurs 2005;21(3):135–6.
5. Finfgeld-Connett D. Concept synthesis of the art of nursing. J Adv Nurs 2008; 62(3):381–8.
6. Paterson JG, Zderad LT. Humanistic nursing. New York: John Wiley; 1976.
7. Williams AM. The delivery of quality nursing care: a grounded theory study of the nurse's perspective. J Adv Nurs 1998;27(4):808–16.
8. Meyeroff M. On caring. New York: Harper & Row; 1971.
9. Finfgeld-Connett D. Qualitative comparison and synthesis of nursing presence and caring. Int J Nurs Terminol Classif 2008;19(3):111–9.
10. MacKinnon K, McIntyre M, Quance M. The meaning of the nurse's presence during childbirth. J Obstet Gynecol Neonatal Nurs 2003;34(1):28–36.
11. Fredriksson L. Modes of relating in a caring conversation: a research synthesis on presence, touch, and listening. Journal of Advanced Nursing 1999;30(5): 1167–76.
12. Farley E. Good and evil: interpreting the human condition. Minneapolis (MN): Augsburg Fortress; 1990.
13. Owens DM. Hospitality to strangers: empathy and the physician-patient relationship. Atlanta (GA): The American Academy of Religion Scholars Press; 1999.
14. Canning D, Rosenberg JP, Yates P, et al. Therapeutic relationships in specialist palliative care nursing practice. Int J Palliat Nurs 2007;13(5):222–9.
15. Levinas E. Totality and infinity: an essay on exteriority. Pittsburgh (PA): Duquesne University Press; 1969. p. 111.
16. Van Kaam A. A personal fulfillment in spiritual life. Wilkes Barre (PA): Dimension Books; 1966. p. 13.
17. Taylor JB. My stroke of insight: a brain scientist's personal journey. New York: Viking; 2008. p. 74–5.
18. Ulrich C, O'Donnell P, Taylor C, et al. Ethical climate, ethics stress, and the job satisfaction of nurse and social workers in the United States. Soc Sci Med 2007;65: 1708–19.
19. Muto S. Caring for the caregiver. Pittsburgh (PA): Epiphany Association; 1996.
20. Rankin EA, DeLashmutt MB. Finding spirituality and nursing presence: the student's challenge. J Holist Nurs 2006;24(4):282–8.
21. Lemonidou C, Papathanassoglou E, Giannakopoulou M, et al. Moral professional personhood: ethical reflections during initial clinical encounters in nursing education. Nurs Ethics 2004;11(2):122–37.
22. Bertolami C. Why our ethics curricula don't work. J Dent Educ 2004;68(4):414–25.
23. Louch, Keith. Formative spiritual glossary of words and phrases. Adrian Van Kaam's Science, anthropology, and theology formation. Pittsburgh: Epiphany Association; 2003. p. 14.
24. Bennett J. Methodological consideration on empathy: further considerations. Adv Nurs Sci 1995;18(1):36–50.
25. Bulechek GM, Butcher HK, Dochterman JC, editors. Nursing interventions classification. 5th edition. St. Louis (MO): Mosby Elsevier; 2008.
26. Moorhead S, Johnson M, Maas M, Swanson E, editors. Nursing outcomes classification. 4th edition. St. Louis (MO): Mosby Elsevier; 2008.
27. The Joint Commission Web site. Available at: http://www.jointcommission.org; 2008. Accessed January 19, 2009.
28. St. Vincent Health. Available at: http://www.stvincent.org. 2008. Accessed January 19, 2009.

29. Gadow S. Existential advocacy: philosophical foundations of nursing. In: Spicker S, Gadow S, editors. Nursing images and ideals. New York: Springer; 1980. p. 90–1.

30. Beckett A, Gilbertson S, Greenwood S, et al. Doing the right thing: nursing students, relational practice, and moral agency. J Nurs Educ 2007;46(1):28–32.

31. Anderson JH, Anderson JH. Nursing presence in a community heart failure program. Nurse Pract 2007;32(10):14–21.

32. Statement on clinical nurse specialist practice and education. 2nd edition. Harrisburg (PA): National Association of Clinical Nurse Specialists; 2004.

33. Iseminger, K. Philosophy as an underpinning for quality of life research PhD dissertation, State University of New York at Buffalo, 1996.

34. DeLashmutt MB. Students' experience of nursing presence with poor mothers. J Obstet Gynecol Neonatal Nurs 2007;36(2):183–9.

35. Snyder M, Brandt CL, Tseng YH. Use of presence in the critical care unit. AACN Clin Issues 2000;11(1):27–33.

36. Roth AJ, Holland J. Psychiatric complications in cancer patients. In: Brain MC, Carbone PP, editors. Current therapy in hematology-oncology. 5th edition. St. Louis (MO): Mosby; 1980. p. 609–18.

37. Gadow S. An ethical case for patient self-determination. Semin Oncol Nurs 1989; 5(2):99–101.

38. Van Kaam A, Muto S. Essential elements of formation anthropology and formation theology: a compilation of complementary considerations. Pittsburgh (PA): Epiphany Books; 2008.

# Thoughtful Nursing Practice: Reflections on Nurse Delegation Decision-Making

Leigh Ann McInnis, PhD, RN, FNP-BC*, Lynn C. Parsons, DSN, RN, CNA-BC

**KEYWORDS**

- Delegation • Decision-making • Nursing practice
- Assistive personnel • Advanced practice nursing
- Licensing • Legislation • Nurse practice act

The complexity of the US health care system continues to escalate. At the same time, uninsured citizens, budget restrictions, and managed care delivery—coupled with advancing medical technologies and an aging citizenry—impact the demand for health care services. In responding to these demands, health care delivery systems are increasingly using a variety of unlicensed personnel to work in patient care areas. In current practice, the licensed registered nurse (RN) plays a significant role in supervising and directing a less skilled workforce and is relied on to make independent decisions regarding the delegation of nursing tasks. Patient care activities and tasks performed 20 years ago by RNs are currently being provided by a workforce that includes assistive personnel (AP), such as medical technicians, licensed practical nurses (LPNs), and other unregulated APs.

As delegators of critical patient care services, professional nurses help to ensure a consistent standard of practice on which the public and the profession continue to rely. This role-related responsibility is especially important given the documented shortage of registered nurses and physicians and the impact this has on the provision of efficient and cost-effective care for patients. As mid-level providers, such as nurse practitioners (NPs), continue to fill this void, it is also vital that nurses understand the responsibilities inherent in the delegation process and implement available guidelines regarding decision making and standards of supervision.

Middle Tennessee State University, School of Nursing, PO Box 81, Murfreesboro, TN 37132, USA
* Correspondence author. Middle Tennessee State University, School of Nursing, PO Box 81, Murfreesboro, TN 37132.
*E-mail address:* lmcinnis@mtsu.edu (L.A. McInnis).

Nurs Clin N Am 44 (2009) 461–470
doi:10.1016/j.cnur.2009.07.002
0029-6465/09/$ – see front matter © 2009 Elsevier Inc. All rights reserved.

## CHALLENGING FACTORS IN HEALTH CARE TODAY

Many factors influence the growing focus on delegation in health care and the increasing use of APs and NPs to augment health care teams. Some of these factors include high patient acuity, competition for health care dollars, rising costs, diminishing reimbursements, increasing numbers of elderly patients, increasing use of technology, and the accelerating pace of change in health care.[1] In addition to these factors, there are concerns regarding staff nurse, nurse faculty, and physician shortages.[2] All of these issues intersect, fueling the need for more nursing services at a time when there are fewer financial and human resources. Delegation is one strategy that health care organizations can use to maximize their current resources.

Although the employment of APs to help fill the void created by the nursing shortage has been shown to decrease costs associated with health care delivery in a variety of settings, certain challenges exist with regard to delegation. For instance, some nurses and some physicians resist delegating and supervising patient care activities performed by APs. Similarly, barriers to effective collaboration between NPs and physicians are well known and include lack of physician knowledge of NP scope of practice, lack of physician knowledge of NP role, unfavorable physician attitude toward NPs, lack of respect, and poor communication.[3] Other issues associated with the delegation process are related to communication patterns, ambiguity in the roles of the delegatee and delegator, lack of experience, and concerns about the scope of responsibility, all of which raise concerns and areas of confusion on behalf of RNs and physicians.

## SHORTAGES OF HEALTH CARE PROFESSIONALS

According to the American Association of Colleges of Nursing report, more than 50% of states experienced nursing shortages in 2000.[1] By 2010, it is expected that 1 million new and replacement nurses will be needed and that by 2015 all 50 states will experience significant shortages.[4] It is evident that over the next few years, the demand for full-time RNs will further exceed the available supply. This growing need for nurses is associated with the retirement of aging RNs, growing demand for nursing care in all health care environments, increasing age of the general and elderly population, technologic advances used in routine and complex care procedures, and rising acuity of hospitalized patients. These factors are driving the overall need for nursing services. The shortage of nurse faculty further complicates this concerning trend and makes it difficult to respond to the demand with an adequate supply.

Similar to their nursing colleagues, physician shortages continue to grow, adding to health care organizations' ability to meet society's need for care. The current nurse and nurse faculty shortage is of critical concern to all stakeholders. In addition to the current nursing shortage, experts believe the supply of physicians will fall short of demand (by 200,000) by 2020.[2] When this impending shortage was reported, nonphysician providers were identified as one factor that might help compensate for the physician shortage. Nonphysician nurse providers include NPs, nurse midwives, clinical nurse specialists, and nurse anesthetists. Although all nonphysician providers play a role in alleviating the physician shortage, NPs are uniquely positioned because of their focus on primary care and health promotion. NP output has held steady over the last several years at 8000. In 2000, there were approximately 90,000 NPs, and that number is expected to rise to 135,000 by 2015.[5] Because of the growing numbers of individuals needing health care services and the increasingly complex technology involved in their care, the increased supply of NPs will not meet the demand for primary care providers nurses, NPs, nurse faculty, physician assistants and physicians.[5–7] The declining number of nurse faculty negatively also impacts the physician and nurse shortages.

## PROFESSIONAL REGULATION
### American Nurses Association

The practice of nursing is based on a social contract with society that acknowledges nurses' rights and responsibilities while upholding their accountability to the public.[8] The American Nurses Association (ANA) defines delegation as the transfer of responsibility for the performance of an activity from one individual to another while retaining accountability for the outcome.[9] The ANA articulates a clear difference between RN and LPN roles. The ANA *Principles for Delegation Paper* offers direction for the RN professional nurse practice role.[9] The ANA document provides definitions for common terms relative to nurse delegation, overarching principles that guide the profession, practice strategies, delegation education, and the ANA delegation model. Information contained within the paper provides the RN with practice strategies when delegating all aspects of patient care to APs.[9]

The ANA model for delegation has 4 major areas for the RN to assess: patient, practice setting, delegatee, and task (**Fig. 1**). Ultimate accountability rests with the RN. He or she must assess the patient and his or her health care needs along with the delegatee's skill set before delegation of any tasks or procedures. The task being delegated to the AP also must have a predictable outcome.

A licensed registered nurse may delegate the responsibility for performing and completing specific nursing care activities to assistants who meet appropriate requirements, usually articulated in a specific job description. The RN holds the assistant responsible for completing appropriately assigned tasks within his or her performance capabilities and specific job descriptions, but the RN remains accountable to the

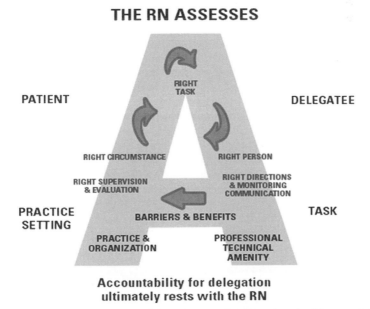

## THE RN ASSESSES

PATIENT

RIGHT TASK

DELEGATEE

RIGHT CIRCUMSTANCE

RIGHT PERSON

RIGHT SUPERVISION & EVALUATION

RIGHT DIRECTIONS & MONITORING COMMUNICATION

PRACTICE SETTING

BARRIERS & BENEFITS

TASK

PRACTICE & ORGANIZATION

PROFESSIONAL TECHNICAL AMENITY

**Accountability for delegation ultimately rests with the RN**

Fig. 1. American Nurses Association delegation model. (*Reprinted with permission from Principles for Delegation*, © 2005 American Nurses Association. All rights reserved.)

profession and its existing standards of care. Similarly, the RN may delegate the "intervention" step of the nursing process to an AP; however, he or she is responsible for supervising the activity and is held accountable for his or her individual actions in the delegation process.

### National Council of State Boards of Nursing

In 2006, the National Council of State Boards of Nursing (NCSBN) and the ANA issued a joint statement on nursing delegation.[6] Although their terminology has some differences, both agencies agree that a professional nurse can delegate tasks to another team member while retaining accountability for the outcome. The NCSBN position paper addressing delegation includes information regarding the delegation decision-making process, common terms, and the role of the RN (delegator) and the delegatee (person receiving delegation).[7,10] The delegation process requires that RNs understand their state nurse practice act, delegator qualifications based on education, skill, and experience, and the delegatee qualifications. Employer/agency job descriptions and individual delegatee performance help the supervising RN determine what can be safely delegated to team members. It is imperative that the RN know their skills and capabilities. It is equally important that they know the abilities of each person assigned to the health care team. The NCSBN model for delegation provides guidance for RNs in their delegation role. The major steps of the model are as follows:

1. Assess the situation: know patient needs, consider the acuity/unit setting, and know the resources available, including supervision
2. Plan for task delegation: identify tasks to be completed and the knowledge required by team members to perform the task; know the skills of team members and any implications for the patient(s)
3. Ensure appropriate accountability: the RN is accountable for the performance of the task and verifies that the delegatee accepts accountability for task completion
4. Supervise task performance: provide direction and expectations for the task to be performed; monitor and intervene if necessary; complete documentation for task completion
5. Evaluate the delegation process: evaluate the patient and delegatee performance and provide feedback to team members
6. Reassess the delegated activity and adjust the care plan if needed[10]

### Five Rights of Delegation

Included in the NCSBN (1995) position statement on delegation are "The Five Rights of Delegation." The five rights are another guide for RNs to use when delegating to team members. The five rights address the right task, right circumstance, right person, right direction/communication, and right supervision in given clinical scenarios (**Box 1**).[10]

The RN uses critical thinking skills and professional judgment when delegating tasks to others. To do this, he or she uses the "Five Rights of Delegation" to determine if the task is appropriate for delegation. These are the right task, under the right circumstances, delegated to the right person, with the right directions and communication, under the right supervision and evaluation.[6]

### State Nurse Practice Acts

State Nurse Practice Acts define the legal boundaries for nursing practice and address the concept of delegation.[7] Some states describe delegation components under the umbrella of supervision. Each state is unique in its ways of dealing with delegation. Effective delegation involves understanding the law for nursing practice, and each state nurse practice act provides nurses with important practice information and guidelines for professional licensure. For example, the *Tennessee State Board of Nursing Position Statement*, Rule 1000-1-.11 describes the RN role relative to delegation under the umbrella of supervision.[11] This rule confirms that RNs must supervise APs by determining which patient care needs can be safely delegated to others and "whether the individual to whom the duties are entrusted must be supervised personally."[11] The Board also interprets "overseeing with authority as requiring on site supervision."[11]

## ADVANCED PRACTICE NURSING AND PHYSICIANS

Health care providers and systems must use all available resources and embrace the concept of delegation to meet the needs of the population. Each health care discipline defines delegation in its unique way; however, these definitions share similarities. The ANA defines delegation as "the transfer of responsibility for the performance of a task from one individual to another while retaining accountability for the outcome."[9] In comparison, the Federation of State Medical boards reports "delegated services must be ones that a reasonable and prudent physician using sound medical judgment

---

**Box 1**
**The five rights of delegation**

• *Right task*

A task that is delegable to a specific patient by a person capable of completing care. The RN must look at the individual patient and his or her condition and know what the expected outcome of care will be. Then a capable delegate is selected. If there is not a capable delegate, the task cannot be delegated.

• *Right circumstances*

The RN must take into account the setting, whether critical care, general surgical unit, or long-term care. Community group homes may be managed by a LPN with RNs available on call. Are appropriate resources available?

• *Right person*

The RN must delegate the right task to the right person to be performed on the right patient. The RN (delegator) must know the role and licensing legislation for LPNs. He or she must know the expectations for each team member outlined in the job description. He or she must know certification guidelines. For example, in some facilities, the RN administering chemotherapy may be required to be certified to give these drugs.

• *Right direction/communication*

The RN must clearly communicate expectations and give specific information on what needs to be done.

• *Right supervision*

The RN gives initial direction and provides periodic inspection of the activity. If the delegatee is new to the team, the RN may want to monitor more closely until the individual's capabilities are conformed. If a nurse is working with an AP who has been on the team for an extended period of time, the RN may choose to periodically inspect at less frequent intervals. The RN who is monitoring and evaluating the work of team members should give feedback often.

*Data from* American Nurses Association (ANA), National Council of State Boards of Nursing (NCSBN). Joint statement on delegation. 2006. Available at: http://www.nccbn.org/Joint_statement.pdf. Accessed December 12, 2008.

would find appropriate to delegate and must be within the defined scope of practice both of the physician and the non-physician practitioner."[12]

## SPECIAL CHALLENGES FOR ADVANCED PRACTICE NURSES

The use of NPs in primary care began in the 1960s in response to an apparent deficit and unequal distribution of direct care physicians. Limited access to health care provided an environment receptive to the NP. Subsequent ebbs and flows in the growth of the physician workforce have been associated with more complex NP/physician relationships, however.[13] When the role of the NP was formalized in the 1960s, physicians wanted NPs to assist them by accepting "delegated tasks." As the role of the NP evolved, NPs demonstrated their ability to function autonomously, and many states responded by increasing their scope of practice.[5] In other states, however, delegation is still used to define the advanced practice nurse (APN) role. Because delegation usually addresses the relationship between physicians and APs or between RNs and APs, it is not an accurate description of the relationship between physicians and NPs. Whether NPs practice independently or as delegatees of the physician, their education and degree hold them accountable to a higher standard.[14]

This lack of standardization has led to confusion over scope of practice, prescribing, and reimbursement for professional services.[3] APNs are thus in a unique position. Delegation for them is a two-pronged issue. On one hand, as a nurse, the APN can delegate tasks to appropriate personnel, such as RNs, LPNs, medical assistants, and APs. On the other hand, in many states, physicians delegate designated services to APNs under their supervision. According to the Pearson Report, 28 states still require some type of physician involvement in APN practice.[14,15] The involvement may include collaboration, supervision, direction, delegation, or authorization of activities.[14]

During a time when predictions indicate an increasing shortage of nurses and primary care providers, state regulations continue to limit scope of practice. Fragmentation of NP practice regulation persists. This state-by-state approach to licensure and scope of practice creates confusion for all stakeholders. In order for delegation to be a successful strategy, physicians must have a clear understanding of NP scope of practice and nurses must understand the scope of practice for APs. Knowing the specific skills that other health care providers possess improves the ability to delegate and supervise while providing safe patient care. A lack of communication, especially related to delegation activity, impairs health care provider relationships.[16] Active communication is the foundation to understanding roles and individual knowledge levels. Regardless of their specific role, all nurses have responsibility for being aware of their professional and state regulations and delegation rules. The role of the nurse as both delegator and delegatee is articulated; however, that information varies from state to state.

## CONGER'S DELEGATION DECISION-MAKING MODEL

The delegation decision-making model developed by Conger is an excellent tool for guiding RNs in delegating to team members.[17] The three-step model outlines the tasks to be completed by the physician, nurse, or agency. The second step involves identifying the problem, whether it is biologic, psychological, or spiritual. In the third step, the RN must evaluate the educational level, know licensing legislation (state nurse practice act), job descriptions, and agency policies, and make a determination of the individual capabilities of the team member being delegated an activity. When these factors have been assessed, the RN makes a delegation decision using sound evaluative criteria (**Box 2**).

Task delegation is performed by physicians and RNs. In the first step of Conger's delegation model, the agency is listed because established procedures mandate certain activities.[17] For example, central venous pressure lines may be changed every 24 hours, peripheral intravenous lines may be changed every 72 hours, and urinary catheters may be cleaned every 8 hours per the agency's established written procedures. This form of delegation is referred to as indirect delegation.

Evaluating patient responses to problems involves RN assessment of the individual. Does the patient have the ability to manage his or her health? Does he or she have knowledge of the disease? Is the patient motivated to complete care procedures? The RN may have an 88-year-old patient who has diabetes and is insulin-dependent and is knowledgeable of the disease, knows how to perform glucose monitoring, and give insulin injections but does not have the visual acuity to draw the correct insulin dose. Conversely, a patient in this same situation may have no visual disturbances but have no desire to perform self-care. These factors impact delegation by the RN.

A trial-and-error approach is not an appropriate learning strategy for delegation skills in the patient-centered environment. Delegation is a skill that can be taught and learned by RNs.[16,18,19] Research by Parsons indicated that as RNs gained

---

**Box 2**
**Delegation decision-making model**

*Patient situation*

- Identify required tasks
    - ordered by the physician
    - ordered by the RN
    - mandated by agency policy
- Identify patient problem
    - biologic
    - psychological
    - spiritual
        - The nurse should assess
            - manageability
            - knowledge (comprehension)
            - motivation (meaningfulness)
- Evaluate most appropriate staff member
    - education
    - job description
    - hospital (agency) policy
    - licensing legislation
    - demonstrated competency

*Data from* Conger MM. Delegation decision-making. Journal for Nursing in Staff Development 1993;9(3):131–5.

delegation knowledge and performed this skill in practice (repetition), their confidence levels for nurse delegation increased.[18] Other research has shown that clinically based educational programs result in increased effectiveness and confidence in delegation.[16,20] Lack of communication can clearly influence attitudes between health care providers. Studies have shown an increase in confidence and job satisfaction in nurses who participate in delegation education and practice the concept using valid delegation tools, such as the delegation decision-making model.[18]

## DISCUSSION

Research supports that many nurses were not taught or even exposed to the concept of nurse delegation decision-making while in their basic nursing programs.[20,21] Although different professional groups and professional nurses may define delegation in different ways, the purpose of delegation remains constant. The purpose of delegation in the practice setting is to complete work safely, efficiently, and correctly.[22] The charge nurse or manager can accomplish efficiency in the practice setting by directing the performance of staff to facilitate patient care outcomes and organizational goals. Delegation can empower team members when done correctly. Proficient delegation also can build confidence and trust among co-workers, enhance communication and teamwork, and build leaders.[18,22]

Delegation is a dynamic process that involves responsibility, authority, and accountability. Each team member is responsible for the completion of accepted tasks. A general guide for RNs is to know individual competencies for each team member. Frequently, job descriptions list tasks that the person holding a certain position can perform. Authority gives the person power to make decisions. Accountability is accepting ownership for the results of task or procedure completion. Accountability cannot be delegated by the RN. Delegation is a critical function for RNs because safe decisions must be made relative to delegation. In many health care environments, APs such as unit clerks, patient care technicians, physical therapy aides, transporters, and phlebotomists perform tasks under the direct supervision of the RN. RNs must assess each team member's capabilities. The safest aspects of care to delegate to unregulated AP are those that do not require critical thinking and have predictable outcomes.[23] Examples of these types of tasks include the following:

- Taking routine vital signs
- Assisting with bathing and oral care
- Passing ice water and meal trays (to patients without swallowing difficulties)
- Changing linens
- Aiding stable, steady patients with walking

Conversely, RNs must not delegate tasks and procedures that require professional judgment, critical thinking, and professional skills. Examples of tasks that may not be delegated include assessment, evaluation of outcomes, medication administration, and care plan development. Nurses in leadership and management roles should not delegate tasks related to employee performance, evaluation, and disciplinary procedures.

Many RNs feel ill-prepared for the role of charge nurse, supervisor, and nurse manager because of their knowledge gap with delegation.[1] Research indicates that a lack of delegation resources in health care settings coupled with inadequate emphasis for teaching delegation in nursing schools has contributed to RNs' inability to safely and confidently direct the workforce. Ultimately, the RN is responsible for tasks and procedures performed by the delegatee. If tasks and procedures are inappropriately delegated and executed, liability lies with the RN.[24]

## BENEFITS OF DELEGATION IN PRACTICE

Successful task delegation optimizes RN time for activities that cannot be delegated. Research shows that the ability to delegate effectively improves satisfaction relative to nurse autonomy (decision-making) on the job and affords promotional opportunities within the organization.[16,19] Quallich[25] concluded that effective delegation improved nurse's job satisfaction, reduced burnout, enhanced time management, and clarified accountability. A study by Curtis and Nicholl[26] confirmed Parsons'[19] finding that effective nurse delegation provides personal and professional advancement in the organization. Nurses who were more productive had additional time for management activities, including conflict management when they were able to delegate effectively. APs reported that effective delegation by the RN improved their skills and knowledge, which enhanced their ability to achieve promotion.[26] These same employees viewed delegation as a positive form of evaluation by the supervisor.[17]

## SUMMARY

To determine the most effective way to implement delegation processes, organizations should evaluate current policies and their success in improving patient care. Initiating or augmenting the use of delegation practices in the health care setting requires a clear and organized approach that incorporates staff education. Nurses must understand their scope of practice, including their state's nurse practice act and professional standards, and the delegation policies of their employer. The American Nurses Association, the National Council for State Boards of Nursing, individual state nurse practice acts, and models for delegation decision-making in the literature provide the RN with safe, objective tools for making delegation decisions. Staff development coordinators in hospital and health care agencies and nurse educators in formal nursing education programs should access these tools to provide information on the policies related to delegation of nursing tasks by registered nurses to unlicensed personnel. Doing so helps to safeguard the authority of the RN to make responsible decisions regarding delegation and ensure that nursing care services have a consistent standard of practice on which the public's trust can be based.

## REFERENCES

1. Kleinman CS, Saccomano SJ. Registered nurses and unlicensed assistive personnel: an uneasy alliance. J Contin Educ Nurs 2006;37(4):162–70 [serial online].
2. Cooper RA. Weighing the evidence for expanding physician supply. Ann Intern Med 2004;141(9):705–14 [serial online].
3. Clarin OA. Strategies to overcome barriers to effective nurse practitioner and physician collaboration. J Am Acad Nurse Pract 2007;3(8):538–48.
4. American Association of Colleges of Nursing [AACN]. Nursing shortage fact sheet. 2008. Last updated September 2008. Available at: http://www.aacn.nche.edu/Media/pdf/NrsgShortageFS.pdf. Accessed January 8, 2009.
5. Cooper RA. New directions for nurse practitioners and physician assistants in an era of physician shortages. Acad Med 2007;82(9):827–8.

6. American Nurses Association (ANA), National Council of State Boards of Nursing (NCSBN). Joint statement on delegation. 2006. Available at: http://www.nccbn.org/Joint_statement.pdf. Accessed December 12, 2008.

7. National Council of State Boards of Nursing [NCSBN]. Working with others: delegation and other healthcare interfaces. 2006. Available at: https://www.ncsbn.org/Working_with_Others.pdf. Accessed December 13, 2008.

8. American Nurse's Association (ANA). Nursing's social policy statement. 1995. Available at: http://www.nursingpower.net/nursing/sps.html. Accessed December 13, 2008.

9. American Nurses Association. Principles for delegation. 2005. Available at: http://www.safestaffingsaveslives.org/WhatisSafeStaffing/SafeStaffingPrinciples/PrinciplesofDelegation.aspx. Accessed January 5, 2009.

10. National Council of State Boards of Nursing [NCSBN]. Delegation concepts and decision-making process: National Council position paper. 1995. Available at: https://www.ncsbn.org/323.htm. Accessed January 8, 2009.

11. Tennessee State Board of Nursing. Position statements. March 2006. Available at: http://www.state.tn.us/sos/rules/1000/1000-01.pdf. Accessed January 5, 2008.

12. Federation of State Medical Boards. Increasing scope of practice: critical questions in assuring public access and safety. Draft report presented at Annual Meeting of FSMB. Phoenix, Arizona, February 2004.

13. US Congress, Office of Technology Assessment. Nurse practitioners, physician assistants, and certified nurse-midwives: a policy analysis. Washington, DC: U.S. Government Printing Office; 1986.

14. Klein TA. Scope of practice and the nurse practitioner: regulation, competency, expansion, and evolution. Topics in Advance Practice Nursing eJournal 2007; 7(3). Available at: http://www.medscape.com/viewprogram/4188_pnt. Accessed January 6, 2009.

15. Pearson LJ. The Pearson report: the annual state-by-state national overview of nurse practitioner legislation and healthcare issues. American Journal of Nurse Practitioners 2008;12(2):9–80.

16. Parsons LC. Delegation skills and nurse job satisfaction. Nurs Econ 1998;16(1):18–26.

17. Conger MM. Delegation decision-making. J Nurs Staff Dev 1993;9(3):131–5.

18. Parsons LC. Building RN confidence for delegation decision-making skills in practice. J Nurs Staff Dev 1999;15(6):263–9.

19. Parsons LC. Nurse delegation decision making: evaluation of a teaching strategy. J Nurs Adm 1997;27(2):47–52.

20. Conger MM. The nursing assessment grid: tool for delegation decision. J Contin Educ Nurs 1994;25(1):21–7.

21. Parsons LC. Delegation decision-making by registered nurses who provide direct care for patients with spinal cord impairment. SCI Nurs 2004;2(1):20–8.

22. Feldman HR, Jaffe-Ruiz M, McClure ML, et al, editors. Nursing leadership: a concise encyclopedia. New York: Springer Publishing Company; 2009:159-51.

23. Williams JK, Cooksey MM. 2004. Navigating the difficulties of delegation. Nursing 2004. Available at: http://findarticles.com/p/articles/mi_qa3689/is_200409/ai_n9424621/pg_1?tag=artBody;col1. Accessed November 30, 2008 [serial online].

24. Pearce C. Ten steps to effective delegation. Nurs Manag (Harrow) 2006;13(8):9 [serial online].

25. Quallich SA. A bond of trust: delegation. Urol Nurs 2005;25(2):120–3.

26. Curtis E, Nicholl H. Delegation: a key function of nursing. Nurs Manag (Harrow) 2004;11(4):26–31.

# Science, Technology, and Innovation: Nursing Responsibilities in Clinical Research

Christine Grady, RN, PhD[a],*, Maureen Edgerly, RN, MA[b]

**KEYWORDS**

- Clinical research • Ethics • Science
- Nursing responsibilities • Human subjects

Clinical research is a systematic investigation of human biology, health, or illness involving human beings.[1,2] The goal of clinical research is to develop or contribute to generalizable knowledge about human health and illness and to test methods that might improve our ability to prevent, diagnose, and treat illness and provide care for patients. Clinical research builds on laboratory and animal studies (preclinical) and often involves clinical trials, which are specifically designed to test the safety and efficacy of interventions in humans. Carefully conducted clinical trials are considered the most reliable way to determine whether therapeutic or preventive interventions are safe and effective for diseases like cancer, HIV/AIDS, and asthma. There are many types of clinical trials, including treatment, prevention, diagnostic, screening, and quality of life, which are defined in **Box 1**.

The benefits of clinical research for society have been significant, yet controversy surrounding it continues to pose profound ethical questions. Nurses are critical to the conduct of ethical clinical research and are involved in research through diverse roles steeped with clinical, ethical, and regulatory challenges. As the volume, diversity, and complexity of clinical research has escalated, the challenges that nurses encounter in the ethical conduct of research have intensified. Examining, understanding, and addressing the unique and complex ethical challenges that face nurses in their various clinical research roles is integral to upholding the moral commitment that nurses make to patients, including protecting their rights and ensuring their safety.

The opinions expressed are the views of the authors and do not necessarily reflect the policy of the National Institutes of Health, the Public Health Service, or the US Department of Health and Human Services.

[a] Department of Bioethics, National Institutes of Health Clinical Center, Building 10/1C118, Bethesda, MD 20892, USA

[b] National Cancer Institute, Medical Oncology Branch, Building 10, Room 12N226, Bethesda, MD 20892, USA

* Corresponding author.

E-mail address: cgrady@nih.gov (C. Grady).

---

**Box 1**
**Types of clinical trials**

Treatment trials test experimental treatments, new combinations of drugs, or new approaches to surgery or radiation therapy.

Prevention trials look for better ways to prevent a disease in people who have never had the disease or to prevent a disease from returning. These approaches may include medicines, vitamins, vaccines, minerals, or lifestyle changes.

Diagnostic trials are conducted to find better tests or procedures for diagnosing a particular disease or condition.

Screening trials test the best way to detect certain diseases or health conditions.

Quality of life trials (or supportive care trials) explore ways to improve comfort and the quality of life for individuals with a chronic illness.

---

Nurses involved in research, as principal investigators (PIs), study coordinators, or clinical trials nurses (CTNs), or as staff nurses caring for patients who are research subjects, have a responsibility to promote the ethical conduct of clinical research. Fulfilling this responsibility requires understanding what clinical research is and knowing what makes it ethical. Only then can nurses determine when to take action for what they believe is right. Consider the following:

Alice is a 42-year-old woman with aggressive cancer that has not responded to previous therapy. She is offered participation in a phase 1 clinical trial with a promising new investigational agent. Alice's nurse knows that the purpose of the trial is to evaluate the safety of the drug and that the possibility of Alice benefiting, through tumor shrinkage or from an increase in length or quality of life, is very small. The nurse is concerned that the PI has not made this clear enough to Alice and that Alice is not well informed about what alternatives are available to her. Respecting Alice's right to make her own decision about study participation, the nurse feels strongly that Alice's informed consent may be compromised. When the nurse raises these concerns, the PI expresses apprehension about confusing Alice. The nurse suggests that a multidisciplinary discussion of the options available to Alice and a plan for ensuring that she understands the options would be helpful for everyone. The PI agrees. The nurse organizes a patient care conference to include the PI, medical fellow, relevant nursing staff, social worker, spiritual counselor, and bioethicist. All agree that it would be helpful if the nurse spent additional time reviewing information about the study with Alice. After a lengthy and engaged discussion with Alice about the study and her options, the nurse asks Alice to explain in her own words what the study is about, what is likely to happen during the study, and what other choices she has besides participation. Much more confident that Alice has a better understanding of the study and is making an informed choice about participation, the nurse offers continued discussion with Alice throughout the study.

To promote valuable clinical research and protect the rights and interests of people like Alice, it is important to be familiar with ways in which clinical research differs from clinical practice. Without an understanding of the purpose of a phase 1 trial or the importance of informed consent to research, the nurse might not have taken any steps to help Alice make an informed decision.

Different phases of clinical trials (outlined in **Box 2**) present different ethical challenges. In the case discussed earlier, for example, the nurse knew that Alice was being invited into a phase 1 trial and believed that understanding the general goals of a phase 1 study was essential to Alice's informed decision.

---

**Box 2**
**Clinical trial phases**

Phase 1. Researchers test an experimental drug or treatment in a small group of people (20–80) for the first time, to evaluate its safety, determine a safe dosage range, and identify side effects.

Phase 2. Researchers test the experimental study drug or treatment in a larger group of people (100–300) to see if it is effective and to further evaluate its safety.

Phase 3. Researcher test the experimental study drug or treatment in a larger group still (1000 or more) to confirm its effectiveness, monitor side effects, compare it to commonly used treatments, and collect information that will allow the experimental drug or treatment to be used safely. Phase 3 trials are usually randomized controlled clinical trials.

Phase 4. Researchers collect additional information after an agent is approved and marketed regarding its risks, benefits, and use in various populations over a longer period of time.

---

## CLINICAL RESEARCH AND CLINICAL CARE

A source of tension for nurses and other health care providers involved in clinical research is differences in goals and methods between clinical research and clinical care.[3] Clinical care encompasses a set of activities designed to promote the welfare and best medical interests of a particular patient. The clinical care provider offers and applies interventions and procedures because they are believed to be safe and effective for the problem at hand. Clinical research, on the other hand, encompasses a set of activities designed to answer a question and generate useful knowledge for the good of future patients or society. Often the rationale for the research is to determine the safety or effectiveness of an intervention for a particular illness. Although individual research participants sometimes do derive medical benefit from research, this is not the primary goal, and some research is not expected to provide any health benefit to participants.[3]

Asking a few individual subjects to assume the burden of research and exposure to risk for the benefit of others creates fundamental ethical tension and ethical obligations in clinical research. These ethical obligations include scientific rigor and social accountability, as well as respect for the rights and welfare of individual participants.[4] In many settings, nurses are ethically responsible for contributing to both the promotion of good science and the protection of the rights and welfare of participants; maintaining the balance requires knowledge, competence, advocacy, creativity, and close working relationships within the research and clinical teams.[5]

**Box 3** provides information about codes of research ethics and other documents that have been developed to provide guidance in conducting ethical research and respecting the rights and welfare of research participants.[6–11] Nurses should be familiar with the major tenets of these codes and know how to access them. Fortunately, educational programs, codes and regulations of research ethics, and other information about clinical research are easily accessible and present opportunities for nurses to learn about the ethical conduct of clinical research. Yet, less than 35% of nurses in one study were familiar with guidelines governing the ethics of research in their department, their facility, or their affiliate university.[11] Although many useful guidelines exist, ethical research is broader and deeper than any code or set of regulations can specify. Ethical research relies on the knowledge, integrity, and judgment of the people involved. As professionals, it is crucial for nurses to have sufficient knowledge to understand clinical research and its ethical requirements and to have the courage to act on this knowledge.

---

**Box 3**
**Codes of research ethics, with URLs**

1. Nuremberg Code http://ohsr.od.nih.gov/guidelines/nuremberg.html

2. Declaration of Helsinki http://www.wma.net/e/policy/b3.htm

3. The Belmont Report http://ohsr.od.nih.gov/guidelines/belmont.html

4. Code of Federal Regulations, Title 45, Part 46, Protection of Human Subjects http://www.hhs. gov/ohrp/humansubjects/guidance/45cfr46.htm

5. Code of Federal Regulations, Title 21, Part 50, Protection of Human Subjects http://www. accessdata.fda.gov/scripts/cdrh/cfdocs/cfcfr/CFRSearch.cfm?CFRPart=50

---

## ROLES AND RESPONSIBILITIES OF NURSES IN CLINICAL RESEARCH

Nurses can be involved in clinical research in many ways. In recent years the volume of and investment in clinical research, in both the public and private sectors, has expanded dramatically.[12] Research is increasingly conducted in nontraditional sites, including contract research organizations and special clinics, private practitioners' offices, and practice research networks. Nurses will encounter clinical research in many settings and will increasingly be called on to offer information to patients, to be involved in recruitment and monitoring, and to advocate for the rights of research participants. The Clinical Center Nursing Department at the National Institutes of Health (NIH) recently launched an initiative called Clinical Research Nursing 2010 to define a specialty practice of clinical research nursing and to work toward a certification process for nurses practicing in clinical research.[13]

The following sections briefly discuss 3 unique nursing roles: (1) the clinical nurse as caregiver of patient-participants before, during, or after participation in clinical research; (2) the nurse as study coordinator or CTN, who works closely with the PI to coordinate all aspects of a study and who may function like a case manager for research participants in the study; and (3) the nurse as PI on a research study, responsible for designing, planning, and conducting clinical research. Each of these roles has its own set of particular ethical challenges.

### Clinical Nurse Caregiver and Research

A clinical nurse might be the first point of contact that a research volunteer has with the clinical research enterprise. The nurse's role could include sharing information about studies for which patients may be eligible, providing general education or information about clinical research, answering questions about specific trials, consulting with clinical research staff, referring patients, and then collaborating with clinical research facilities on the participant's care. A clinical nurse or clinical research nurse might also be employed by a health care facility that conducts clinical research and therefore may, as a staff nurse, directly care for individuals who are participating in a clinical trial. Nurses sometimes support study implementation within the context of clinical care in dedicated clinical research settings, such as the NIH Clinical Center, or in clinical research units located in academic medical centers across the country.[13] The nursing care provided to research participants takes into account study requirements and the collection of research data, as well as clinical indications and patient care needs. The clinical nurse might, for example, administer investigational medications, perform a detailed clinical assessment, collect research samples, and communicate with the research team regarding observed results. Additional or specialized nursing care may be necessitated by the response of the participant to a study intervention.

The clinical nurse might have more direct contact with individual research participants than other members of the research staff. The relationship of the nurse with the research participant might start before or end after the clinical trial. For example, in a community practice setting, a nurse might care for a patient for several years before the patient is referred to a clinical trial at an urban research center. The community practice nurse will hopefully maintain a supportive relationship while the patient is participating in the trial and resume the primary care relationship when participation is complete. Good communication between the research center and the referring office helps to minimize possible misinformation or frustration that could affect the patient's experience.

Since a clinical nurse could influence a patient's decision about participating in a clinical trial, the nurse should understand what research is and what the particular trial is about. For example, consider patients who participated in a clinical trial for testicular cancer. This trial involved investigational chemotherapy along with computerized tomographic monitoring and 2 laparotomies, 1 pre- and 1 posttreatment, to measure response to the chemotherapy. Not understanding the need for the second laparotomy, the nurse was concerned that it subjected the patient to unnecessary and possibly objectionable risk. Only after asking questions and learning about the purpose and details of the study was the nurse able to appreciate the need for the second laparotomy and fully support the patient in this trial. Several studies have shown a relationship between familiarity with research methods and procedures and nurses' acceptance of and support for research.[14–16]

The clinical nurse, providing care to a patient participating in a clinical trial, may not have any involvement in the research other than direct and frequent access to the patient and his or her family or support system. As the caregiver, however, the nurse might be the first to recognize and communicate adverse events, lack of adherence with study requirements, or the effect of participation on the patient-volunteer's disease and psychosocial situation. The nurse may be in the best position to notice an adverse event cluster, especially when it includes common symptoms like fatigue, anorexia, and arthralgias, and can help to distinguish such adverse events from natural disease progression. Clinical nurses caring for research participants need accurate and up-to-date information about the disease under study and the particular objectives, interventions, procedures, and ongoing findings of the clinical trials that involve their patients. The research team should make such information available to clinical nurses and help them recognize their role in communicating critical data to the research team. Collaboration, interest, and participation of clinical nursing staff are essential to the successful and ethical conduct of clinical research.

### CTN/Study Coordinator

Many nurses function as study coordinators, research coordinators, or clinical trial nurses (CTN). These roles may vary from organization to organization, but there are elements common to many settings. Some nurses who transition from a clinical position to that of a study coordinator or CTN, initially experience a sense of isolation and lack of support in these roles. In addition, they are often surprised by conflicts with clinical nurses or a perceived lack of interest on their part.[17]

The primary responsibility of the CTN is to safeguard the integrity of the study while managing study participants. Each study has specific requirements that must be adhered to, in order for the results to be valid and interpretable. The CTN works to ensure that the study requirements are met consistently, while balancing the safety and rights of research participants. Research nurse coordinators or CTNs are usually responsible for study coordination and data management, which often includes responsibility for managing subject recruitment and enrollment and for eligibility screening. CTN's provide education and counseling regarding informed consent, and in some cases, obtain informed consent. They ensure consistency of study implementation, accurate collection of specimens, monitoring of subjects throughout the study, and study drug accountability. The CTN also ensures collection, management, and integrity of data and compliance with regulatory requirements and reporting, among other things.[18] Research nurse coordinators are often hired by and report to a PI for support of a specific study or group of studies. A CTN or research nurse coordinator is responsible for the study and is an advocate for it and for the participant, both as subject and as patient.

The role of CTN has been recognized as a distinct subspecialty by some professional organizations, such as the Oncology Nursing Society (ONS). The ONS has published an extensive Manual for Clinical Trials Nursing[19] and has a special interest group that publishes educational modules about clinical trials and a regular newsletter for CTNs.[20]

### Nurse PI

Nursing research, to develop a scientific basis for practice, is critical to evidence-based quality care for patients. Nurses as PIs are responsible for designing, implementing, and analyzing research, aiming to expand the science base for care. Similar to any clinical researcher, the nurse PI has many ethical obligations with respect to clinical research, including asking a clinically or scientifically useful question and designing the study, methods, and procedures in a rigorous and feasible manner. PIs must also fairly identify appropriate research participants to be invited into the research, minimizing the research risks and maximizing potential benefits; they must send the proposal through the appropriate levels of independent review, obtain the informed and voluntary consent of participants, and carefully monitor and respect the participants' rights and welfare throughout the study.[4]

Nurses who are researchers face all the ethical challenges inherent in conducting research. In addition, nurse researchers can confront situations that involve tension or intrinsic conflicts between their roles as clinicians and researchers. In the course of research, for example, a nurse researcher may become aware of, or receive a request for, a health care intervention that a patient may need. Patients should not be expected to appreciate the distinction between the nurse as caregiver and the nurse as researcher.

When and how a nurse researcher intervenes depends on the study design, the relationship the researcher has with the participant, and, importantly, the nature of and immediacy of the patient's need. Researchers have an obligation to intervene when there is an acute, serious, or life-threatening situation. For example, a nurse studying the relationship between diet and hypoglycemia in teenagers would intervene if a teen became syncopal because of hypoglycemia.

In other cases, however, intervening may be incompatible with answering an important research question that the nurse researcher is studying. A nurse surveying teens on their sexual behavior, for example, might appropriately plan not to provide interventions, education, or referrals, at least until the survey questions had been completed. In designing any study, the nurse researcher should anticipate the kinds of interventions that might be needed and carefully plan how to respond to patient needs during and at the end of the study, including knowing what referral and care options are available.

Decisions about how to intervene and respond to a patient may be particularly challenging in qualitative research, in which the relationship between the researcher and the research participant can influence the direction and the integrity of the data.[21,22] For example, one study concluded that nurses need more research education and team and management support when conducting research, with opportunities to debrief after encountering mixed role expectations in the field.[23]

## BALANCING ADVOCACIES

Regardless of the position that a nurse holds in clinical research, a recurrent challenge is balancing the various advocacies that stem from the role or roles that the nurse plays, advocacies that can and sometimes do come into conflict. These are outlined in **Table 1**, and include advocacy for the individual as patient, advocacy for the individual as research subject, and advocacy for the research itself.[24]

The professional role of the nurse as patient advocate, supported by nurses' intuitions, may result in an instinctive approach to conflicts from that perspective. The American Nurses Association Code for Nurses describes the nurse as an advocate for the patient.[25] Similarly, the American Association of Critical-Care Nurses identifies patient advocacy as an integral component of critical care nursing and states unequivocally that "[a] nurse's primary ethical obligation is to patients" and notes that "…the professional nurse should advocate the highest quality of health care for patients and

**Table 1**
**Nursing advocacies in clinical research**

| Role & Advocacy | Patient Advocacy | Research Participant Advocacy | Research Advocacy |
|---|---|---|---|
| Clinical nurse | The clinical nurse's primary role is care and advocacy for the patient. | As patient advocate, the clinical nurse also has an important role in making sure that the patient knows about appropriate research opportunities and has needed information about the study and his or her rights as a research participant. | The clinical nurse may have a critical role in performing procedures consistent with the research plan, and/or reporting symptoms and side effects that may be important to the research question. |
| CTN | Having been trained as a patient advocate, the CTN keeps in mind what is best for the patient when considering the patient as a possible research participant. | The CTN has a critical role in ensuring that participants are recruited in a responsible manner, are well-informed about the study and that their rights and welfare are protected. | The CTN is a pivotal member of the research team, working closely with or for the PI to successfully and ethically conduct the research. |
| Nurse PI | The nurse as PI should be prepared for the possible conflict between what is best for the patient and what is best for the research. | The nurse as PI is responsible for protecting the rights and welfare of research participants in his/her study and seeking support from others for the same. | The nurse as PI is responsible for rigorous and quality research design and implementation, conducted in an ethical manner. |

families... [and] must judge between the requirements of the study and the changing needs of the patient."[26]

Patient advocacy is integral to nursing in any setting. Nurses generally spend more time with patients than do other care providers; therefore, they are in a primary position to assess and evaluate whether research participation is or continues to be consistent with a patient's best interests, values, and preferences. Occasionally, the nurse may advocate a reconsideration of the patient's participation in a research study based on changes in the patient's condition or the patient's choices, even though such advocacy could conflict with the expectations of the research team.

The nurse working in any capacity with research participants should act as an advocate for the research participant. This requires some knowledge about participants' rights and the types of protection in place for human subjects in clinical research. For example, the nurse acts as an advocate for research participants by helping to ensure that they understand the study and what they are being asked to do, receive the information needed to make informed decisions before and during the study, and are aware of their right to withdraw without penalty.

The nurse also has a role in advocating for the research itself. Clinical research is important for advancing health care and our understanding of health for the benefit of patients now and in the future. Whether the nurse is primarily a caregiver, a CTN, or an investigator, there is a responsibility to advocate and support the goals of research and contribute responsibly to the validity and integrity of the study. Each of these advocacies is important and requires the nurse to recognize and balance them, emphasizing the appropriate priority at any given time. The primacy of each of these advocacies shifts depending not only on the nurse's role but also on the specifics of the situation and requires informed and careful judgment. Consider the following examples:

BK works at a community clinic as a primary care nurse and has known some of the clinic patients for many years. Dr. Smith, the physician who runs the clinic, recently became an investigator for a clinical trial of a new drug for mild to moderate depression. A sign was hung in the clinic advertising the study and Dr. Smith has already mentioned it to several patients. BK has reviewed the study and thinks it is worthwhile and well designed. BK also knows that Dr. Smith is excited about being part of the trial, is counting on the financial support from the pharmaceutical company for the study, and sincerely hopes the drug will be successful. One morning, Mr. N asks BK if he should join the study. During the discussion, Mr. N mentions that he likes and trusts Dr. Smith and thinks that joining the study might make Dr. Smith happy. BK is conflicted because Dr. Smith has asked her to help recruit patients and she knows that Mr. N might be eligible for the study, but Mr. N's reasoning makes her uncomfortable. BK's responsibility to advocate for the study seems in conflict with her responsibility to act as an advocate for Mr. N.

BK explains her discomfort to Mr. N and assures him that she and Dr. Smith are committed to taking care of him in the best way possible regardless of whether he participates in the study. She emphasizes that participating in the study is his choice and one that should be carefully considered. They plan a future appointment and in the meantime agree that Mr. N should look over the study information, take time to think about it, and discuss it with his wife. He mentions that his cousin is a doctor and he will probably also ask her for some advice. BK has acted as an advocate for Mr. N as both a patient and a potential research subject.

### Consider Another Example

KB is a CTN for a phase 2 clinical trial of an investigational treatment for a progressive neurologic disorder. A patient, who does not speak English and has no health insurance, comes to the research facility for possible enrollment in the trial. The trial requires 5 inpatient treatments, each cycle with additional monitoring for toxicity. The patient's husband has stopped working to care for his wife. They have received an eviction notice from their landlord. The CTN evaluates the patient for eligibility and is concerned that she will not be able to comply with the demanding protocol schedule or have adequate resources (phone, transportation, and a stable home) to participate safely. The research team proposes a meeting with the patient and with her permission also invites her husband and their adult sons. The situation and concerns are explained. The adult children, who had been shielded from information about the severity of their mother's illness, offer to move both parents into one of their homes and care for them, providing food, phone, and transportation to help their mother complete the treatment protocol.

The CTN is also concerned that the patient, in reality, has few options and is potentially vulnerable because of the language barrier and lack of insurance. Treatment within the clinical trial is free, and she is clear that this is an important reason for her interest. The CTN arranges for an interpreter to provide assistance when discussing informed consent, a social worker to explore options for health care coverage, and an ethics consultation to impartially assess the patient's decision and reasoning.

In this situation, the CTN advocates the study (by seeking to enroll eligible subjects that can adhere to the study plan), acts as an advocate for a possibly vulnerable subject (by arranging assistance in translating the consent discussion, in exploring alternative options, and in impartially assessing the decision), and acts as an advocate for a patient who is facing a difficult situation and needs treatment for her disease (by involving the family in a supportive problem-solving discussion about the immediate and long-term challenges).

### Or This Example

RN is the research coordinator at her institution for a large multi-center clinical trial studying treatment of men with prostate cancer. Participants are elderly men, some are quite ill, and they are randomized into 1 of 3 different treatment arms. RN is responsible for recruiting participants at her site and for seeing them at the clinic each week to collect blood samples, vital signs, and symptom data. RN has been the research coordinator for multiple studies and understands the need for monitoring participant safety and for collecting important data along the way. However, she is concerned that in this study, coming to the clinic each week presents a significant burden for some of the elderly ill participants. Because this is a multi-center study, she is also aware that the PI at her site is unlikely to want to vary the study in ways that might change the design. She meets with the PI to explore 2 possible alternatives for reducing participant burden that could be compatible with the study design: a small cadre of nurses could visit the participants in their homes to collect blood and vital signs, and the frequency of the blood collection could be reconsidered if there were alternatives to a clinic visit for monitoring participant safety. In this situation, RN is exercising advocacy for the study participants, by trying to reduce burden, and for the study, by proposing alternative methods of obtaining needed data that won't compromise the design.[27]

### One Final Example

NR is the PI of a study investigating environmental factors believed to influence the adjustment and well-being of mothers and infants within the first 2 weeks postpartum. As part of the study, NR meets the mothers before they are discharged from the hospital and obtains their consent to make once-weekly visits to their home. At each home visit, NR administers a questionnaire to the mothers and observes the interaction between mother and baby and the circumstances in the home. On one scheduled home visit, NR finds Sue's baby unattended and crying uncontrollably. Sue, the mom, is asleep in the next room and apparently has not heard the baby. NR wants to understand and record this finding but also feels compelled to attend to the baby and to investigate why Sue is not responding to the baby's crying. After picking up the baby, NR attempts unsuccessfully to wake Sue. Seeing an empty pill bottle by Sue's side, NR calls 911 for emergency assistance and asks the neighbors how to contact Sue's husband. NR went to Sue's home as a researcher, but intervened as a nurse and advocate for both Sue and her baby.

## SUMMARY

The nurse's obligation to the patient includes conducting and supporting research in a manner that benefits society by generating useful knowledge, while respecting and protecting individuals who contribute to the endeavor. Morally responsible nursing consists of recognizing and responding to situations in the most ethical manner that promotes quality patient care. Knowing, understanding, and addressing the ethical challenges that complicate clinical research are essential functions for all nurses in the diverse roles that are critical to the process.

## REFERENCES

1. Grady C. Ethical principles in clinical research. Chapter 2. In: Gallin J, Ognibene F, editors. Principles and practice of clinical research. 2nd edition. Burlington (MA): Elsevier; 2007. p. 15–26.
2. Grady C. Clinical trials in the Hastings Center bioethics briefing book for journalists, policymakers, and campaigns. New York: Hastings Center; 2008. p. 11–4.
3. National Commission for the Protection of Human Subjects of Biomedical and Behavioral Research. The Belmont report: ethical principles and guidelines for the protection of human subjects of research. Washington, DC: US Government Printing Office; 1979.
4. Emanuel E, Wendler D, Grady C, et al. What makes clinical research ethical? JAMA 2000;283(20):2701–11.
5. Grady C. Clinical research: the power of the nurse. Am J Nurs 2001;101(9):11.
6. Nuremberg Code. Available at: http://ohsr.od.nih.gov/guidelines/nuremberg.html.
7. World Medical Association. Declaration of helsinki. Available at: http://www.wma.net/e/policy/b3.htm. Accessed May 14, 2009.
8. U.S. National Commission for Protection of Human Subjects in Biomedical and Behavioral Research. The belmont report. Available at: http://ohsr.od.nih.gov/guidelines/belmont.html. Accessed May 14, 2009.
9. U.S. Code of Federal Regulations Title 45 Part 46, Protection of Human Subjects. Available at: http://www.hhs.gov/ohrp/humansubjects/guidance/45cfr46.htm. Accessed May 14, 2009.
10. U.S. Code of Federal Regulations Title 21 Part 50, Protection of Human Subjects. Available at: http://www.accessdata.fda.gov/scripts/cdrh/cfdocs/cfcfr/CFRSearch.cfm?CFRPart=50. Accessed May 14, 2009.
11. Alt-White A, Pranulis M. Addressing nurses' ethical concerns about research in critical care settings. Nurs Adm Q 2006;30(1):67–75.
12. Tufts Center for the Study of Drug Development. Outlook. 2009. Available at: http://csdd.tufts.edu/InfoServices/OutlookReports.asp. Accessed May 9, 2009.

13. NIH Clinical Center Department of Nursing. Clinical Research Nursing 2010: Background and Overview. Bethesda: NIH Clinical Center; April 2009.
14. Albers LL, Sedler KD. Clinician perspectives on participation in research. J Midwifery Womens Health 2004;49(1):47–50.
15. Smirnoff M, Ramirez M, Kooplimae L, et al. Nurses' attitudes toward nursing research at a metropolitan medical center. Appl Nurs Res 2007;20(1):24–31.
16. Tanmet J, Lochhaus-Gerlach J, Lam M, et al. The effect of staff nurse participation in a clinical nursing research project on attitudes toward, access to, support of and use of research in the acute care setting. Can J Nurs Leadersh 2002; 15(1):18–26.
17. Spilsbury K, Petherick E, Cullum N, et al. The role and potential contribution of clinical research nurses to clinical trials. J Clin Nurs 2008;17(4):549–57 [Epub 2007 Apr 5].
18. Ehrenberger H, Lillington L. Development of a measure to delineate the clinical trials nursing role. Oncol Nurs Forum 2004;31(3):E64–8.
19. Klimaszewski A, Baum M, Deininger B, et al. Manual for clinical trials nursing. Pittsburgh (PA): Oncology Nursing Society; 2008.
20. Oncology nursing society, SIG virtual communities. Clinical trial nurses special interest group. Available at: http://clinicaltrial.vc.ons.org. Accessed May 2, 2009.
21. Jack S. Guidelines to support nurse-researchers reflect on role conflict in qualitative interviewing. Open Nurs J 2008;2:58–62.
22. Hewitt J. Ethical components of researcher-researched relationships in qualitative interviewing. Qual Health Res 2007;17:1149–59.
23. Beale B, Wilkes L. Nurse researcher: always a researcher, sometimes a nurse. Collegian 2001;8(4):33–9.
24. Davis A, Hull S, Grady C, et al. The invisible hand in clinical research: the study coordinator's critical role in human subjects research. J Law Med Ethics 2002; 30(3):411–9.
25. American Nurses Association: Code of Ethics for Nurses with Interpretive Statements. Washington, DC: American Nurses Publishing; 2001.
26. American Association of Critical Care Nurses. Ethics in critical care nursing research. Available at: http://www.aacn.org/WD/Practice/Content/Research/ethics-in-critical-care-nursing-research.pcms?menu=Practice. Accessed May 5, 2009.
27. Veatch R, Fry S. Case studies in nursing ethics. Philadelphia: Lippincott; 1987. p. 244, case 91.

# Care and Meaning in War Zone Nursing

Ernestine (Tina) Cuellar, RN, PhD[a,b,*]

**KEYWORDS**

• Nurse • Military • War • Stress • Caring • Nursing • Austere

## HISTORICAL RELATIONSHIP BETWEEN NURSES AND WAR ZONES

Contemporary nursing is a complex moral process, built on the lives, accomplishments, and motives of its famous historical exemplars, and shaped by scientific discoveries, medical innovations, and societal movements. Philosophically, it can be viewed as the outcome of a great humanitarian awakening to the needs of others and to the diverse forms of caring, healing, and helping that mark its professional ideology. From a practical viewpoint, contemporary nursing is a responsible action, centered on the needs of human beings and the application of knowledge and experience to improve the lives of others. Although nursing currently enjoys a respectable and authoritative position in society, the historical path by which it attained its current status as a trusted health profession is unique. Indeed, for about 300 years from the mid sixteenth century until 1858, nursing lacked any aura of respectability. Charles Dickens' satirical character Sairey Gamp depicted the prevailing view of nineteenth century nurses as easily bribed, drunken women of low or no morals.[1,2] Many nursing historians have described early nineteenth century hospital nurses as tough, socially marginal women, characteristics that were attributed by some to the thankless work that they were called on to perform.[3–5] Before her interventions, both Florence Nightingale[6] and her contemporaries described untrained nurses of her time as drunkards,[5] attributing this to the reputation that nursing had as a menial, badly paid occupation that required no training.[6] These depictions of the conduct, character, and social conditions of nurses are difficult to reconcile with the virtuous practice that characterizes the profession today, especially in situations where safeguarding the lives and well-being of others requires sacrifice and courage.

The opinions herein are those of the writer, and do not necessarily reflect the views of the US Air Force or the Department of Defense.
[a] University of Texas Medical Branch, School of Nursing, 301 University Boulevard, Galveston, TX 77555–1032, USA
[b] Mental Health Department, 433 Aeromedical Staging Squadron, Lackland Air Force Base, San Antonio, TX, USA
* Corresponding author. University of Texas Medical Branch, School of Nursing, 301 University Boulevard, Galveston, TX 77555–1032.
*E-mail address:* ehcuella@utmb.edu

Nursing is an ancient calling, but the period of its greatest growth is that of the last hundred years. This growth is stimulated by new forms of knowledge to improve the care of the ill, whether they reside in homes, hospitals, ambulatory clinics, or on the battlefields of the world. For centuries, nurses have been present in every type of crisis situation, including various plagues, pandemics, and wars. In a variety of ways they have participated in every war of the last century, serving near the front lines in the troubled areas of the world, and behind the scenes in hospitals and evacuation units.

Throughout history, nurses have provided care for soldiers in war zones, and Florence Nightingale is credited with revolutionizing the care of those wounded in war. Despite extraordinarily difficult personal and social conditions she managed to change the disreputable image of nurses during the Crimean War. In 1854, British soldiers were dying in large numbers from injuries and illness while the Catholic sisters were saving the lives of French soldiers in the Crimea.[1,7,8] Nightingale's petition to go to Crimea coincided with the British government's request that she provide nursing care and save the lives of British soldiers in that war zone.[1,7,8]

In 1858, Nightingale was appointed Superintendent of Female Nurses in Scutari.[7,8] She selected 38 nurses including ten Roman Catholic Sisters, 2 Protestant nurses, 8 Sisters of Mercy, and 6 Sisters of St. John's house, as well as 14 nurses from various hospitals.[1,2,8] The members of the contingent of nurses were considered controversial because of the religious majority—most contentious was the inclusion of Catholic Sisters—for there was fear that the religious nurses would be less concerned with healing wounds than healing the spiritual needs of the soldiers.

In the Crimea, Nightingale found soldiers with dirty dressings, living in cold, unsanitary conditions with leaking ceilings, abundant rodents, and poor food.[2,7,8] Despite the fact that the Nightingale contingent was greeted with antipathy by the medical staff,[1,8-10] she created a legacy to nursing by emphasizing prevention through improving health and sanitary conditions, and is credited with significantly reducing the death rate.

After 2 years in the war zone, Nightingale was supervising 125 nurses who provided the foundation for the resurrection of respect for nurses. She is credited with saving thousands of lives by introducing cleanliness and infection control. Unfortunately, while in the Crimea Nightingale became ill.[2,8] On her return to England, although her health remained precarious, she continued to work from her home. In 1873, funds from British soldiers and their supporters were used to found the first professional nursing school, as conceptualized by Nightingale, at St. Thomas' in London.[2,8]

During the past century nurses have served as caregivers for United States military personnel in every major theater of war. While Nightingale was establishing professional nursing in Great Britain, Dorothea Dix was being appointed Superintendent of Women Nurses in the Army[11] and author Louisa May Alcott was volunteering as a nurse during the American Civil War (1861–1863). Alcott published a book, and a quote from her writing epitomizes the experiences of nurses from the Crimean War to the present, describing her experiences during the civil war as:

> My first (sic) three days' experience had begun with a death, and... a somewhat abrupt plunge as superintendent of a ward containing forty beds... the amputations were reserved till the morrow... their (the men's) fortitude seemed contagious, and scarcely a cry escaped them, though I often longed to hear a groan from them ... (much later) more flattering...was the sight of... rows of faces... lighting up with smiles of welcome, as I came among them, enjoying that moment heartily...with a motherly affection for them all.[1]

Following nurses' participation in World War I (1914–1918), a notable distinction for nursing was the establishment of a section for Army and Navy Nurses at Arlington National Cemetery.[11] In World War II (1939–1945), 59,000 nurses served in the US Army, and 200 nurses died, 16 as result of enemy fire. Nurses were Japanese prisoners of war (POWs)[12] and in a bombardment of an Army hospital by Germans, 3 nurses were killed while another 3 were wounded. Nurses served on hospital ships and in the Philippines, providing care for wounded and ill soldiers and sailors, as well as local women and children.[11,13]

Nurses in the Korean War worked in a frigid and hostile environment while living in austere environments. Operating room nurses worked 18-hour shifts wearing men's uniforms, and in one day flight nurses assisted in evacuating almost 4000 wounded Marines and Army soldiers from Korea. The Vietnam War, which ended in 1973, marked the first time in United States history that nurses had been assigned to combat areas. Nurses worked long and arduous hours under threat of personal injury or death to bring compassion and caring to soldiers who were nearly always mortally wounded.[14]

Nurses have participated in both Gulf Wars. The first Gulf War (1990–1991) was short, and during that time nurses cared for Iraqi prisoners of war, as well as local women and children.[12] Hundreds of soldiers, marines, and airmen lived because nurses and other health care providers placed themselves in harm's way to ensure the welfare of soldiers. The ongoing second Gulf War, which has been characterized as the first major war of the twenty-first century, began in March 2003. Each year hundreds of military medical personnel (nurses, physicians, and medical technicians) volunteer or are sent to war zones and humanitarian missions throughout the world. This article focuses military nurses in Iraq to provide care to US military personnel, coalition forces, civilian contractors, Iraqi citizens (primarily women and children), and detainees. Although nurses have described a sense of personal satisfaction for the care they provided, there is evidence that some nurses have felt unprepared for war zone nursing.[15]

## IN HARM'S WAY

From the time of antiquity, caring individuals have placed themselves in harm's way, calming the dying, easing pain, and providing calm to those in distress. As battles rage across many fronts, nurses continue to answer the call to help. These individuals serve as flight nurses, surgical nurses, teachers, and leaders, with the common goal of protecting others and preserving an allegiance to country, self, and profession. Professional nurses have faced uncomfortable working and living conditions while providing care and treatment in war zones. For many, the most important reward for living in discomfort and facing the possibility of injury or death is the appreciative response of the wounded or ill soldier, marine, sailor, or airman. Thoughts are often voiced by military personnel when they see the medic or arrive at the hospital or hospital ship. These comments embody the feelings of soldiers, sailors, and airmen toward the nurses and other health care personnel who risk their lives to ensure that the soldiers receive medical care.[16]

*I was naked on my back on the bed… the pain chewed at me… I didn't know what was wrong… "Hi, Marine." I looked up into the beautiful brown eyes of a navy nurse wearing a starched white uniform. "Frostbite?" I asked. Frostbite could mean amputation. It scared the hell out of me….The navy nurse bent down beside me and held my hand. Her voice was soft, yet firm, "You'll be fine. It will all work out." I was safe. I fell asleep.[16]*

The situations described repeat throughout the twentieth and now into the twenty-first century. No matter where the war zone is located, soldiers' attitude toward nurses, medical technicians, and physicians is timeless—merely seeing and knowing the existence of nursing and medical personnel creates a sense of safety in the experience of the wounded. Without question, serving in a war zone and deliberately placing oneself in harms' way is stressful. The nature and source of stress, including complex ethical dilemmas facing military nurses providing care to patients in a war zone and the similarity of nurses' experiences as they travel throughout the world to uncomfortable environments and dangerous places to provide compassionate care for soldiers is a genuine challenge. The rewards, however, are unquestionable.

> … There was a sense of accomplishment that nurses felt when going through this deployment [sent to a war zone]… there is no real way to describe the interaction between nurses and soldier patients. Patients are wearing the same uniforms as the nurses and it's a different feeling from what nurses usually feel with patients. There is a bond that is not there generally with civilian patients. Although you maintain a professional interaction, there is a closer connection while caring for a soldier, a Marine, a sailor, or an airman in pain and distress…the nurses felt rewarded by the patients' appreciation of what was done.[15]

### NURSING IN IRAQ: THE AUSTERE ENVIRONMENT

The sights, sounds, and smells of a war zone assault the senses and nurses in a war zone may be overwhelmed by sensory overload. There is also information overload as a massive amount of input has to be processed in the first few days. In Iraq, personal risk to military medical personnel is also an environmental factor. When nursing personnel arrive in the war zone, they are immediately faced with constant threats from mortar and rocket grenades. The AFTH consisted of 25 Army tents therefore nurses must wear protective body armor weighing 30 to 50 pounds and may at times be required to wear arms while providing care (**Fig. 1**). Sensory overload (the stimuli of the war zone, adjustment factors, and the amount of information that nurses receive) diminishes the ability to process information and make clear decisions, and may intensify the risk.[17] Turbulence in the war zone has been described as stress both in the work and living environment leading to increased vulnerability for nurses and physicians.[17]

A newly arrived nurse must care for young military personnel with multiple serious injuries, care for severely injured women and children, and care for injured hostile detainees. These activities cause major stress as nurses adjust to being in an austere work environment in a new country.[18–24] Other significant stresses that affect nurses while deployed have been reported in several studies, including the effect of traveling thousands of miles to a different environment, leaving loved ones, and feeling a sense of isolation from the familiar (**Fig. 2**).[15,25–28]

### THE NATURE OF THE INJURIES TREATED

Body armor protects the soldier's trunk from injury[29] therefore in Iraq, injuries to the extremities or the head and neck were the most frequently seen. Insurgents target the ears, nose, and throats of soldiers and civilians with bombs filled with shrapnel and toxins. Surgical interventions are required for injuries including complex facial lacerations, facial burns, and also for exploration of the neck for penetrating trauma, tracheotomy, and tympanic puncture.[30–33]

Injuries by explosive devices create polytrauma, which accounted for the largest number of patients cared for in the intensive care unit (ICU). One nurse recounted an example of a typical shift change report:

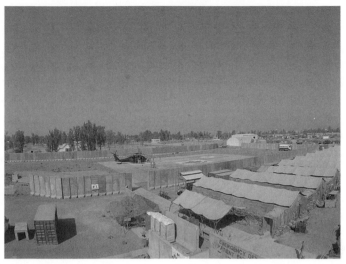

**Fig. 1.** Until August 2007 when a permanent facility was completed, the Air Force Theater Hospital (AFTH) was housed in 25 Army canvas tents. The AFTH had approximately 60 inpatient beds, 18 critical beds, 8 emergency trauma beds, and 3 operating suites.

*Unknown Iraqi male of unknown age who arrived by Blackhawk helicopter last night after being injured in an explosion. He returned from the operating room ... following a celiotomy and right thoracotomy with intercostal artery repair, right central jugular vein repair, right chest tube inserted for a hemothorax, liver laceration packed, abdomen remains open with wound VAC (vacuum-assisted closure) device in place. Other injuries included a right lower and a right upper extremity amputation (and) penetrating fragmentation wounds, contusive organ blast effects, traumatic brain injury, traumatic amputations, complex soft tissue injuries, gunshot wounds, and second and third degree burns.*[31,34–36]

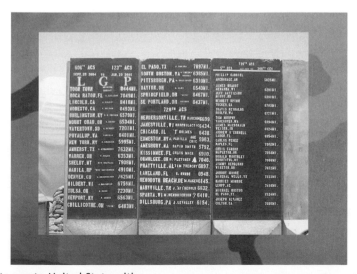

**Fig. 2.** Distances to United States cities.

A source of great pride for military nurses in Iraq was the 97% survival rate, as well as that of 2000 critically ill medically evacuated patients, in whom the death rate was less than 1% for patients who received care at the Air Force Theater Hospital (AFTH).[31,34–36] At the AFTH, patients were treated and stabilized for transport to a higher level of care. Critically injured patients were aeromedically transported from the AFTH within hours of surgical repair and stabilization. An en route "flying ICU" was used for the critically injured patient.[30,32,37–39] Patients received one-to-one in-flight care from a critical care nurse, a respiratory therapist, and a physician (**Fig. 3**).[32,34,35,37,39]

Death in the war zone affects everyone. Nurses as well as physicians, medical technicians, chaplains, and other ancillary personnel made it a point to provide "presence" for a dying patient. One anecdote described the death of a young man with burns over 90% of his body. Medical personnel from all disciplines—nursing, medicine, pharmacy, physical therapy, and the chaplaincy—sang *Amazing Grace* to the young man until he took his last breath,[40] exemplifying the credo of "being with" a patient in the war zone.

> *...the tenacity of the staff at the hospital was probably the most rewarding ... to see the best of people come out and their dedication and their selflessness to take care of the wounded... that was the most meaningful and rewarding... throughout my life it's probably something that I'll look back on positively.*[41]

### CIVILIANS: WOMEN AND CHILDREN

Injured Iraqi women and children were often admitted to the AFTH, including the ICU. Iraqi civilian patients had longer lengths of stay than American or Coalition soldiers, who were aeromedically evacuated to Landstuhl Regional Medical Center within 4 to 12 hours postoperatively.[31,32] The disposition of Iraqi citizens was complicated as there was limited ability for the AFTH to arrange transfer to Iraqi health care facilities,[31,32] although Army Civil Affairs officers often facilitated patient transfers and outpatient follow-up care in Baghdad.[42]

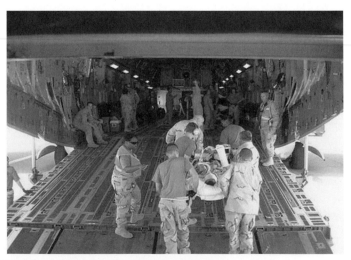

**Fig. 3.** Transporting ICU patients from Iraq to Germany.

Nurses found ways to advocate for the health care and welfare of local women and children. For example, one nurse wrote home and asked her community to send care packages with common items such as toothpaste, toothbrushes, soap, and deodorant, as well as coloring books, and small games for the children (B. Burton, personal communication, February 18, 2008). She was able to hand out several thousand boxes to patients. In another example of nursing altruism and advocacy, books were collected from universities in Texas that were then transported to nursing schools in Iraq.[43]

## DETAINEES

In addition to upholding moral and ethical commitments of the nursing profession, AFTH nurses are required to adhere to the Geneva Convention, providing comparable care to all patients brought to the hospital. Because of this, US and Coalition soldiers, civilians, and enemy combatants were provided equal treatment.[30,44] Nurses identified situational and ethical stress while caring for injured detainees, especially for those detainees who were responsible for severe injuries incurred by American soldiers, Coalition forces, and local women and children. At times, the injured detainees were verbally abusive to female caregivers making it difficult for nurses to maintain their healing and helping attitudes. These stressors have also been described by nurses in other wars such as World War II, the Korean War, and the Vietnam War.[15,25–27,44]

Mental preparation for the verbal abuse accompanied by abusive gestures was necessary to prepare nurses for the conflict resulting from threats to their personal safety. The internal struggle related to resolving ethical dilemmas required nurses to take risks that affected their satisfaction with their jobs and their commitment to patient advocacy.[45] It was exceptionally difficult for nurses to care for orphaned Iraqi children and women who were seriously injured by improvised explosive devices (IED) or gunfire perpetrated by the detainees.

## THE PHYSICAL ENVIRONMENT

The heat and dust were a shock on arrival in the war zone.[46,47] For example, the environment in Kuwait has been described as "…pretty much what you expect: white, hot, and sandy. To simulate the Kuwaiti experience, turn a hair dryer on high and stick it on your eyeball. And throw sand on yourself."[46] Temperatures higher than 130°F (54.4°C) were reported, and adjusting to the heat while wearing flack vests required acclimation.[46] Nurses were physically stressed, working in temperatures of 110°F (43.3°C) or greater, while droning air conditioners operating at full capacity added to the stressful environment.[15]

Lack of personal privacy was identified as increasing feelings of personal vulnerability because there was no place where an individual could be alone.[15] Additional stress was related to long working hours with little time off, inclement weather, frequent mortar attacks, loud noise emanating from alarms, living close to the flight line, and hearing planes land and take off, as well as the din of aeromedical evacuation helicopters bringing newly wounded patients to the AFTH (**Fig. 4**).[15,25,27,28,41]

## CONCERN FOR PERSONAL SAFETY

Multiple studies of nurses deployed in World War II and Vietnam described concerns for personal safety in the work and living environment of a war zone.[25–28] In Iraq, daily mortar attacks created challenges in the work environment.[33,47] For example, it was

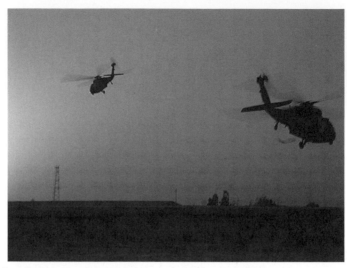

**Fig. 4.** Medivac helicopters bringing the wounded to the AFTH.

not unusual for mortar-round explosions to occur while walking to work or rockets exploding meters from living quarters.[31] There have been limited deaths among physicians, nurses, and medical technicians assigned to the AFTH; however, medical technicians who are combat medics are at an increased risk of death or injury. Wearing body armor is uncomfortable and although it increases the physical workload, it is necessary.[29] Body armor and helmets are worn by medical personnel in the hospital tents while providing patient care whenever there was a threat of mortar attack.[29,30]

### RESILIENCE IN THE FACE OF DANGER

A common thread noted in qualitative reports by military nurses working in a war zone is their resilience in the face of multiple stressors.[14,25,27,44,48] Resilience is defined as the ability to recover quickly from setbacks or problems, and to develop and strengthen protective factors to cope with environmental and societal stressors.[49–52] Addressing the challenges nurses encounter in the war zone has been ameliorated by their commitment to the military and to each other.

> The most meaningful rewarding thing about this deployment (for me) was the support of the nurses for other nurses and the feeling that patients really, really cared about what the nurses provided for them.[40]

Appropriate measures to mitigate stresses of nurses before deployment to extreme environments such as a war zone are imperative. Programs that successfully train people to manage extreme stress by desensitization include employing repetitive practice exposure before actual exposure.[30,53,54] Practice and rehearsal create memories that provide automatic and repeatable responses even under pressure.[55]

### SUMMARY

Military nurses in the war zone deliver patient care while working in austere conditions, and are under threat of personal danger. Six components of military nurses' competence to practice in austere environments include (a) clinical nursing competence, (b) operational competence, (c) personal, psychological, and physical readiness, (d) soldier/survival skills, (e) leadership and administrative support, and (f) group integration and identification.[56]

The nature and sources of stress in the war zone are environmental, situational, and emotional. At various times, nurses find their aims as nurses in conflict with dimensions of the situations in which they find themselves. Nursing in the military requires a range of cognitive competencies and emotional skills, all of which are employed under conditions of uncertainty, scarcity, and stress. Multiple ethical dilemmas affect patient care, and nurses employ diverse means to manage the conflicting situations they confront. A validating factor enhancing the role and self-confidence of the nurse in the war zone is patient care.[15] For military nurses, learning to cope with multiple stressors while providing optimal patient care reinforces Nightingale's view of nursing as "What nursing has to do …is to put the patient in the best condition for nature to act upon him."[57]

The same could be said of nurses themselves—that military nursing has to focus on the needs of the nurse who deliberately places herself or himself in harm's way—that others might be less vulnerable to the ravages of war. Nurses in the military have a unique opportunity to heed the call of humanity to improve health and well-being, to use their skills not only to calm and ease the suffering, but to safeguard the lives of others.

## REFERENCES

1. Jamieson E, Sewall M. Trends in nursing history: their relationship to world events. Philadelphia: W.B. Saunders Company; 1940.
2. Jensen D. A history of nursing. St Louis (MO): The C.V. Mosby Company; 1943.
3. Kalisch PA, Kalisch BA. The advance of American nursing. Boston (MA): Little, Brown; 1978.
4. Melosh B. The physician's hand: work culture and conflict in American nursing. Philadelphia: Temple University Press; 1982.
5. Reverby SM. Ordered to care: the dilemma of American nursing 1850-1945. Cambridge (MA): Cambridge University Press; 1987.
6. Cook E. The life of Florence Nightingale. New York: MacMillan; 1942.
7. Dossey B. Florence Nightingale. Springhouse (PA): Springhouse Corporation; 1999.
8. Woodham-Smith C. Florence Nightingale. New York: McGraw-Hill book Company, Inc; 1951.
9. Hines D. Black women in white. Indianapolis (IN): Indiana University Press; 1989.
10. Carnegie M. The path we tread: blacks in nursing. Philadelphia: J.B. Lippincott Co; 1986.
11. Sterner D. In and out of harm's way: a history of the navy nurse corps. Seattle (WA): Peanut Butter Publishing; 1996.
12. Smolenski M, Smith D, Fanney J. A fit, fighting air force: the air force nursing service chronicle. Washington, DC: Office of the Surgeon General; 2005.
13. Littleton M, Wright C. Doc: heroic stories of medics, corpsmen, and surgeons in combat. St Paul (MN): Zenith Press; 2005.
14. Sarnecky M. A history of the U.S. Army Nurse Corps. Philadelphia: University of Pennsylvania Press; 1999.
15. Cuellar E. Nursing in the combat zone: psychological implications of patients with traumatic injuries. Presented at the Annual Meeting of the Association of Rehabilitation Nurses, Oct 2–7, 2007, Washington, DC.

16. Omori F. Quiet heroes: navy nurses of the Korean War, 1950–1953, far east command. St. Paul (MN): Smith House Press; 2000.
17. Menzies I. Nurses under stress. Int Nurs Rev 1960;7:9–16.
18. Brailey K, Vasterling J, Constans J, et al. PTSD symptoms, life events, and unit cohesion in U.S. soldiers: baseline findings from the neurocognition deployment health study. J Trauma Stress 2007;2:495–503.
19. Carson M, Paulus L, Lasko N, et al. Psychophysiologic assessment of post traumatic stress disorder in Vietnam nurse veterans who witnessed injury or death. J Consult Clin Psychol 2006;68:890–7.
20. Maguen S, Turcotte D, Peterson A, et al. Description of risk and resilience factors among military medical personnel before deployment to Iraq. Mil Med 2008;173:1–9.
21. Stevenson M, Schloes R, Dremsa T, et al. Readiness estimate and deployability index for Air Force nurse anesthetists. Mil Med 2007;172:36–9.
22. Susarick AL. Life events in health care providers before and during the Persian Gulf War deployment: the USNS Comfort. Mil Med 1999;164:75–82.
23. Turner B, Turse N, Dohrenwend B. Circumstances of service and gender differences in war-related PTSD: findings from the National Vietnam Veteran readjustment study. J Trauma Stress 2007;20:643–9.
24. Wynd C. A proposed model for military disaster training nursing. Online J Issues Nurs 2006;11:5.
25. Norman E. We band of angels: the untold story of American nurses trapped on Bataan by the Japanese. New York: Random House Inc; 1999.
26. Baker R, Menard S, Jones L. The military nurse experience in Vietnam: stress and impact. J Psychol 1989;45:736–44.
27. Freedman D, Rhoads J. Nurses in Vietnam: the forgotten veterans. Austin (TX): Texas Monthly Press; 1987.
28. Pflantz S. Work stress in the military: prevalence, causes, and relationships to emotional health. Mil Med 2002;167:877–82.
29. Ricciardi R, Deuster P, Talbot L. Effects of gender and body adiposity on physiological responses to physical work while wearing body armor. Mil Med 2007; 172:743–8.
30. Smith K. Critical care nursing in an austere environment. Crit Care Med 2008; 36(Suppl 7):S297–303.
31. Berkowitz G. Otolaryngologists on the front lines. ENT Today 2007;2:12–4.
32. Fecura S, Martin C, Martin K, et al. Nurses' role in joint theater trauma system. J Trauma Nurs 2008;15:170–3.
33. Holt GR. An otolaryngologist as flight surgeon: one doctor's experience in operation Iraqi freedom. ENT Today 2007;2:13.
34. Johannigman J. Disaster preparedness: it's all about me. Crit Care Med 2007; 33(Suppl 7):S22–8.
35. Johannigman J. Maintaining the continuum of en route care. The evolution of military trauma and Crit Care Med: application for civilian medical care systems. Crit Care Med 2008;36(Suppl 7):S377–82.
36. Mason PE, Eadie E, Holder A. Prospective observational study of United States Air Force critical care aeromedical transport team (CCATT) operations in Iraq. Journal of Emergency Medicine 2009;11(1), in press.
37. Grathwohl K, Venticinque S. Organizational characteristics of the austere intensive care unit: the evolution of military trauma and critical care medicine; applications for civilian medical care. Crit Care Med 2008;36(Suppl 7):S275–83.
38. Venticinque S, Grathwohl K. Critical care in the austere environment: providing exceptional care in unusual places. The evolution of military trauma and Crit

Care Med: applications for civilian medical care systems. Crit Care Med 2008; 36(Suppl 7):S284–92.

39. Blackbourne L. Combat damage control surgery. Scientific Reviews 2008; 36(Suppl 1):S306–10.

40. Cole E. Paper presentation: R3: Readiness, resilience, rejuvenation presented at 114th Annual Meeting of the Association of Military Surgeons of the United States; Nov 10–16, 2008, San Antonio, TX.

41. Cuellar E. Paper presentation: Ethical dilemmas and stress: Resiliency in deployed military nurses presented during Annual Meeting of the American Holistic Nurses Association; June 6–9, 2007, Lake Tahoe, California.

42. Ferguson M. Civil affairs. Sustainer Magazine 2006; Available at: http://www.3esc.army.mil/news/sustainer/SustainerSpecialEditionFINALsmall.pdf. Accessed date July 11 2008.

43. Brannon B. Department of the Air Force presentation to Committee on Appropriations Subcommittee on Defense. 2004. Available at: www.sg.af.mil/sharedmedia/document/AFD. Accessed date June 17 2009.

44. Duncan R, Pansoy C, Towe L, et al. Grace under fire. Nursing 2005;35:62–4.

45. Gilligan C. In a different voice. Cambridge: Harvard University Press; 1982.

46. Irwin M. From clinical nurse III to first lieutenant: nursing at the Abu Ghraib prison hospital. Am J Nurs 2005;105:79–81.

47. Cotton S. The best worst job I've ever had. Am J Nurs 2007;107:86–7.

48. Norman E. Women at war: the story of 50 military nurses who served in Vietnam. Philadelphia: University of Pennsylvania Press; 1990.

49. Flach F. (1997, 2004). Resilience: discovering a new strength at times of stress. New York: Ballantine Books; 2009.

50. Almedom A. Resilience, hardiness, sense of coherence, and post-traumatic growth: all paths leading to "Light at the end of the tunnel"? Journal of Loss and Trauma 2005;10:253–65.

51. Tusaie K, Dyer J. Resilience: a historical review of the construct. Holist Nurs Pract 2004;18:3–10.

52. Lambert CE, Lambert VA. Psychological hardiness: state of the science. Holist Nurs Pract 1999;13:11 9.

53. Beard C, Wilson J. Experiential learning: a best handbook for educators and trainers. 2nd Edition. Philadelphia: Kogan Page; 2007.

54. Kolb D. Experiential learning. Englewood Cliffs (NJ): Prentice Hall; 1984.

55. Caine G, Caine R, Crowell S. MindShifts: a brain compatible process for professional development and the renewal of education. 2nd Edition. Tucson (AZ): Zephyr Press; 1999.

56. Reineck C. Individual readiness in nursing. Mil Med 1999;164:251–5.

57. Nightingale F. Notes on nursing: what it is and what it is not. Philadelphia: J.B. Lippincott; 1946.

# Perspectives on Transcultural Care

Dana Bjarnason, PhD, RN, NE-BC[a],*, JoAnn Mick, PhD, RN, AOCN, NEA-BC[b],
Julia A. Thompson, PhD, RN, CIP[c], Elizabeth Cloyd, MBA, RN, NEA-BC, FACHE[d]

**KEYWORDS**

- Transcultural • Caring • Diversity • Culture
- Moral and ethical reasoning

Culture has been defined as the thoughts, communications, actions, customs, beliefs, values, and institutions of racial, ethnic, religious, or social groups.[1] An ideal culture suggests attributes that are most desired or preferred or the wished for desires of a group. A culture of nursing refers to the learned and transmitted lifeways, values, symbols, patterns, and normative practices of members of the nursing profession of a particular society.[2] In the culture of health care, these norms refer to the way information is received, rights and protections are exercised, and even what is considered to be a health problem.[1] Clearly, health care is a cultural construct, central to the effective delivery of health care services. In nursing, respect for persons has continuously been maintained as a core ethical principal of professional practice. To serve the unique and diverse needs of patients in the United States, it is imperative that nurses understand the importance of cultural differences by valuing, incorporating, and examining their own health-related values and beliefs and those of their health care organizations, for only then can they support the principle of respect for persons and the ideal of transcultural care.

## TRANSCULTURAL NURSING

More than 5 decades ago, nurse theorist Madeleine Leininger began exploring culture concepts from the field of anthropology and care concepts from nursing, forming the construct of culture care.[3] Leininger defined transcultural nursing as a humanistic and scientific area of formal study and practice in nursing focused on differences and similarities among cultures with respect to human care, health, and illness and is based on

[a] Ben Taub General Hospital, Quentin Mease Community Hospital, 1504 Taub Loop, Houston, TX 77030, USA
[b] Nursing Research & Clinical Outcomes, Harris County Hospital District, 2525 Holly Hall, Houston, TX 77054, USA
[c] Research & Sponsored Programs, Harris County Hospital District, 2525 Holly Hall, Houston, TX 77054, USA
[d] Harris County Hospital District, 2525 Holly Hall, Houston, TX 77054, USA
* Corresponding author.
E-mail address: dana_bjarnason@hchd.tmc.edu (D. Bjarnason).

Nurs Clin N Am 44 (2009) 495–503
doi:10.1016/j.cnur.2009.07.009
0029-6465/09/$ – see front matter © 2009 Elsevier Inc. All rights reserved.
nursing.theclinics.com

cultural values, beliefs, and practices.[4] Culture in American hospitals has been shaped by nursing, and Leininger discussed several major reasons for examining this phenomenon. Of particular relevance to the idea of the culture of nursing is Leininger's postulation that nurses need to understand and appreciate inherent differences and similarities not only locally but also regionally, nationally, and worldwide.

Although it is clear that values, norms, and standards differ in nursing globally, the moral commitment that nurses make to patients includes upholding cherished human virtues, such as sympathy, compassion, faithfulness, and truth telling. There is a connection between Leininger's postulation that caring is the central and unifying domain for nursing knowledge and practice and her belief that professional nursing care embodies scientific and humanistic models of helping or enabling patients to maintain a healthy condition for life or death.[5]

## CULTURAL DIVERSITY AND THE NURSING WORKFORCE

Understanding and responding to diversity in health care is especially challenging in the United States because of America's increasingly multicultural society and the different ethnic, religious, and personal values not only of patients but also of health care providers. Globalization, immigration, and nursing shortages have created complex issues related to patient care delivery and the nursing workforce. Globalization is reflected in the increasing interaction and integration among people and governments and is driven by international trade, investment, and commerce.[6] Immigration has significantly affected and radically changed the composition of the population and the workforce in the United States. In the midst of these changes, nursing shortages that began in the middle of the last century have led to the employment of increasing numbers of foreign-born and foreign-educated registered nurses (RNs), which now represent a considerable segment of the practicing US nurse workforce. The growing US nursing workforce dependence on foreign-born RNs is evidenced by statistics that indicate that 37% of total RN employment growth is attributed to the rapid growth of employment of foreign-born nurses.[7]

Although the problem of minority underrepresentation in nursing is particularly acute (the percentage of nurses from racial and ethnic minorities grew only from 7% in 1980 to 12% in 2000), this lags significantly behind the proportion of minorities in the general population, which is approximately 30%.[8] Complicating this finding is the fact that although 15%[7] of nursing full-time equivalent positions in the United States are foreign-born minorities, they do not necessarily represent the face of America.

Racial and ethnic population statistics from the 2000 national census estimated that whites comprised 75.1% of the US population, whereas 12.3% were black or African American and 3.6% were Asian. Of the total population, 12.5% represented Hispanics or Latinos of any race.[9] In contrast to national population statistics, the racial/ethnic makeup of the RN workforce practicing in the United States is 84.9% white, 3.2% black or African American, 1.7% Asian, and 1.2% Hispanic, with the remaining 9.6% comprised of all other races/ethnicities.[10] Gender and age/generational diversity further complicate factors related to cultural diversity in the nursing workforce. Although 49.1% of the US population is male compared with 50.9% female,[9] 93.8% of nurses employed in nursing are women, compared with 6.1% who are men.[10] Demographic trends and low recruitment during health care workforce restructuring in the 1990s have resulted in a nursing workforce that represents 4 generations and is more skewed toward older workers than the general workforce.[11–13]

## NURSING'S EVOLVING POSITION ON DIVERSITY

Nursing's voice in valuing diversity is evidenced in the evolution of the American Nurses Association "Code of Ethics for Nurses." Since the Code's inception in 1893, the profession of nursing's ethical stance has reflected a value in people and relationships. At that time, nurses pledged to "devote myself to the welfare of those committed to my care."[14] By 1940, nurses provided public statements that "honesty, understanding, gentleness, and patience should characterize all acts of the nurse" and that "the nurse has a basic concern for people as human beings... [and] respect for [the] religious beliefs of others."[15] In 1950, nursing first introduced language that substantially addressed the issue of justice in the health care setting, proclaiming that "the need for nursing is universal ...[and that] professional nursing service is...unrestricted by considerations of nationality, race, creed, or color."[15]

Nurses' commitments were strengthened in the 1976 revision of the code when the connection between people, relationships, and diversity were first introduced in ethical statements describing perspectives of human dignity and respect for persons. The new provision recognized the uniqueness of each individual, requiring the nurse to provide care "with respect for human dignity...unrestricted by considerations of social or economic status, personal attributes, or the nature of health problems."[15] Further changes to the code in 1985 clarified, redirected, and sometimes altered the nuance of the original provisions, demonstrating a shift from the character virtues of nurses to the rights of patients and principles of professional nursing conduct. Although in 1976, the code mandated quality nursing care as a right of all citizens, in 1985 citizenship was irrelevant to any consideration of access to or distribution of nursing health care services.[16]

The most recent revisions to "The Code of Ethics for Nursing" occurred in 2001. The value of diversity continues to be a strong assertion, as evidenced by the first provision, which states that "the nurse, in all professional relationships, practices with compassion and respect for the inherent dignity, worth, and uniqueness of every individual, unrestricted by considerations of social or economic status, personal attributes, or the nature of health problems."[17] In addition to the code of ethics, the American Nurses Association bolstered nursing's position relative to the moral and ethical treatment of patients and the importance of understanding the relationship between nurses and patients when it published a position statement that was released in October 1991 entitled "Cultural Diversity in Nursing Practice." This document offers guidance regarding the need to understand—among other things—the influence of the cultural background of the nurse on care delivery, with particular emphasis on the need to understand that the nurse-patient relationship is influenced by three distinct interactions: the culture of the nurse, the culture of the patient, and the culture of the setting.[18]

## NURSING'S SOCIAL POLICY STATEMENT AND DIVERSITY

Nursing's social policies offer another strong example of the commitment that US nurses make to honoring diversity. Last updated in 2003, "Nursing's Social Policy Statement" is a fundamental document that describes the articulation of nursing and its social framework and obligations. Simply, it is the expression of the social contract between the public and the nursing profession in the United States.[19] The current document was derived from the 1980 landmark document "Nursing: A Social Policy Statement" and the 1995 document "Nursing's Social Policy Statement." The social policy statement provides a framework for nursing's understanding of the profession's relationship with society and the obligation to the recipients of nursing care.

The statement articulates values and assumptions that characterize the value of diversity, including that human experience is contextually and culturally defined and that the interaction between the nurse and the patient occurs within the context of the values and beliefs of both.[19]

## NURSING'S PROFESSIONAL REGULATION AND DIVERSITY

In addition to the code of ethics and the social policy statement, nursing has defined its professional regulation (as opposed to legal regulation) in a 2004 document entitled "Nursing Scope and Standard of Practice," which outlines 6 standards of practice that describe a competent level of nursing care. Themes that consistently arise and are integral to the practice of professional nursing include providing culturally and ethnically sensitive care and communicating effectively.[20] Although these themes represent just a fraction of the actions required of RNs, their connection to the need to understand and value diversity—not only of their patients, but within the profession—is clear. The standards reflect nursing's values and priorities and are the authoritative statements for which nurses are accountable.[20]

## US WORKFORCE RESPONSE TO DIVERSITY

Visible differences in the workforce related to age, languages, religions, race, ethnicity, sexual orientation, abilities, disabilities, levels of education, skills, and experiences have increasingly appeared as demographics have continued to shift in the United States.[21] Although diversity in the workplace has brought many benefits to organizations, it also has created many challenges.[22] As technology, growth, globalization, and socioeconomic advances continued to effectively connect diverse cultures, industries and professions began to initiate efforts to manage increasingly diverse workforces by implementing management strategies such as cultural awareness, sensitivity, diversity training, and cultural competencies.[23] In health care, diversity training has helped to increase awareness of differences and promoted sensitivity and attentiveness to interactions between faculty and staff. Health care providers began to focus on understanding how and why different belief systems, cultural biases, ethnic origins, family structures, and other culturally determined factors influenced the illness experience, treatment decision making, adherence to medical advice, and response to treatment and how these factors led to differences in care outcomes.[24] Cultural competencies were developed to assure required knowledge, skills, attitudes, and behaviors to provide optimal health care services to persons from a wide range of cultural and ethnic backgrounds.

As organizations were attempting to address diversity with training, however, management researchers began to identify that rapid and significant increases in work force diversity would result in communication problems, potential for increased organizational conflict, and a high degree of value incongruence among members of the work force immigrating to the United States from a variety of culturally diverse countries.[25] Researchers proactively identified that without learning and understanding how to work together, the productivity of new recruits and existing employees would be less than optimal. Failure to address cultural aspects of teamwork could lead to low morale, ineffective communication, and interpersonal conflict. Initially, assimilation was the predominant management strategy used to integrate foreign recruits into the existing workforce. Expectations for newly hired employees to forgo prior knowledge and experiences often suppressed their ability to express themselves genuinely in the workplace setting, thus denying significant parts of their lives in a social context and causing increasing frustration.[26] Assimilation into the dominant organizational culture began to show negative consequences for individuals and organizations. A greater focus emerged on management of workplace conflict, including addressing the topic of horizontal violence. Employers began to provide educational opportunities for workers to acquire skills to more effectively deal with interpersonal conflict.

To better address employee dissatisfaction and interpersonal conflict in the workforce, the current frame of reference has begun to change from an ethnocentric view of adoption of "our way is the best way" to a more culturally relative perspective of using the best of a variety of practices.[27] Assuring opportunities for all employees to openly contribute their ideas and passion to accomplish an organization's mission can support goal achievement and improved business outcomes. Beyond the acknowledgment of diversity by culture, an organization can achieve increasing respect for the range of knowledge and experiences offered by employees with diverse backgrounds.

## CULTURAL COMPETENCE AND THE VALUE OF DIVERSITY

The first step in the evolution toward organizational cultural competence is to align objectives of the initiative with the organization's mission, vision, and values and with applicable regulations, guidelines, and accreditation requirements. The mission/vision, values, and philosophy of a health care organization must establish a high regard for diversity by embracing the provision of culturally sensitive care as a consistent platform for operations, including that every individual has the right to be treated with dignity and respect. In health care organizations, nurses bring their personal cultural heritage and the cultural and philosophic views of their education into the organizational setting. The literature consistently suggests that cultural competence begins with individual self assessment.[28] To understand that there are multiple equally justifiable culturally determined values, systems, and behaviors, nurses must first be aware of and understand their own set of values.[29] Cultural competence must become an inherent part of the organizational culture.

*"…the customary way of thinking and behaving that is shared by all members of the organization and must be learned and adopted by newcomers before they can be accepted into the agency…a combination of assumptions, values, symbols, language, and behaviors that manifest the organization's norms and values."[30]*

In 2002, the Commonwealth Report defined cultural competence in health care as "the ability of systems to provide care to patients with diverse values, beliefs, and behaviors, including tailoring delivery to meet patients' social, cultural, and linguistic needs."[31] Cultural competence is one of the key elements thought to reduce disparities in health care, and it must be achieved at the organizational, systemic, and provider levels. A competency program can assist an organization to establish effective communication systems between different cultures. Examination of the cultural variations that make a difference in health care can generate opportunities to transition a culturally diverse environment into a collaborative workforce. To be successful, a cultural competency program requires a strong commitment at the organizational level and should identify manageable and concrete goals, outline operational plans to meet those goals, and establish management accountability and oversight mechanisms.

The assessment of cultural competence in nursing may be accomplished through the use of various tools. For example, the National Center for Cultural Competence at Georgetown University captures a wide range of information in its "Cultural Competence Health Practitioner Assessment," which includes 6 subscales: (1) values and belief systems, (2) cultural aspects of epidemiology, (3) clinical decision making,

(4) life cycle events, (5) cross-cultural communication, and (6) empowerment/health management.[32] The American College of Healthcare Executives, the American Hospital Association, the National Center for Leadership, and the Institute for Diversity in Health Management combined efforts to develop a research-based diversity and cultural competence tool that can be used for a baseline evaluation of a health care organization's diversity management performance. The tool "Strategies for Leadership: Does Your Hospital Reflect the Community It Serves?"[33] can be used to evaluate the diversity and cultural proficiency of an organization and identify existing activities and practices and those that may need to be implemented.

Employee satisfaction surveys offer 1 approach to evaluate the outcomes of a cultural competence program. Other methods include maintenance of records of appeals, complaints, grievances, and lawsuits, differentiated by the ethnicity of the complainant and guaranteeing "whistle-blower" immunity to employees who draw attention to practices, actions, or policies that are not culturally competent.

## CULTURALLY COMPETENT CARE

The Commonwealth Report also identified many barriers to the delivery of culturally competent care that are relevant to a community, including lack of diversity in health care leadership and workforce, systems of care poorly designed for diverse patient populations, and poor cross-cultural communication between providers and patients.[31] The inability of a provider to understand socioeconomic differences may lead to patient noncompliance, which can affect health outcomes. Health care leaders can take action to deal with these disparities, including development of patient assessment tools that explore cultural values, alternative medicine, and family roles in illness. At the organizational level, interventions to address these barriers include fostering the hiring and promotion of a diverse work force and working to understand the needs of the community. At the systemic level, evaluating the structure of the entire health care delivery system to include culturally appropriate programs, disease management programs, and educational materials is imperative. At the clinical competence level, health care providers must be equipped with knowledge of health beliefs of different cultures.

In order for optimum patient care to occur, patients must trust their providers. Effective communication is critical to building trust in the patient/provider relationship and in team relationships. Trust comes from the ability to communicate, understand, and be understood. Ideally, staff communicate effectively in the language of the patient. The availability and deployment of on-site, in person, or telephonic interpreters is critical. Written materials also should be available at appropriate reading levels and in the language that the patient and family can understand.

In health care, challenges to effective communication may be exacerbated by culturally distinctive dialect, speech patterns, or colloquialisms of patients and/or providers. Providing elocution classes to the workforce is one strategy for managing employee communication concerns. Actions that can assist providers to effectively communicate with patients include providing access to a medically trained translator when the provider does not speak the patient's language, assessing patients' baseline understanding when communicating by encouraging patients to ask questions, and using plain language without medical jargon. Highlighting 1 to 3 important points the patient needs to remember, providing important instructions in written format in the patients' preferred language, and providing educational materials, pictures, and drawings whenever possible also promote effective communication and enhance understanding.[34]

National standards on culturally and linguistically appropriate services are available from the Office of Minority Health.[1] There are 14 culturally and linguistically appropriate services standards that focus on language to improve understanding between patient, family, and providers and address culturally appropriate care. The instruments used to gather information from patients must be broad enough to capture information that encompasses culturally specific beliefs about health and illness (eg, use of herbal remedies and family roles in illness). Knowledge of these basic tenets allows for care planning that embraces a patient's belief system in the treatment plan.

## TOWARD A TRANSCULTURAL IDEAL

In view of the increasing range of diversity within the care-receiving and care-providing segments of society in the United States, it is more important than ever to focus on understanding and addressing the impact of diversity and its relationship to patient care. Now more than ever, health care leaders are charged with understanding and managing diversity to maintain a healthy, productive, and respectful work environment. By aligning organizational objectives to appreciate the diverse nature of health care providers and patients, the work and care environments are enriched. By addressing cultural diversity in health care, employers can keep employees engaged and motivated, thereby maximizing patient safety and productivity.

Although multiple generations and cultures are working together, further increasing the diversity of the nursing workforce is necessary to successfully expand health care access for underserved populations.[35] The development of a diverse nursing workforce will help to expand health care access for the underserved, foster research for neglected societal needs, and enrich the pool of managers and policymakers to meet the needs of an increasingly diverse US population.[36,37] To build a diverse workforce that meets the needs of a diverse population, nurse leaders need to continue to assess their existing workforce culture and systems to identify barriers and strategies to effectively attract and retain culturally diverse employees, enhance recruitment/hiring processes, and create positive work environments. Focusing on diversity and the culture of nursing in formal programs has inherent benefits. It assists newcomers in understanding dominant, recurrent, and patterned features of nursing, serves as a valuable historical guide to past, current, and future change,[2] and reinforces the moral commitment that nurses make to patients, which mandates the need to understand nursing care practices and appreciate the differences and similarities among all nursing cultures.

## REFERENCES

1. US Department of Health and Human Services. 2001. National standards for culturally and linguistically appropriate services in health care. Available at: http://www.omhrc.gov/assets/pdf/checked/finalreport.pdf. Accessed June 4, 2009.
2. Leininger M. The tribes of nursing in the USA culture of nursing. J Transcult Nurs 1994;6:18–22.
3. Murphy SC. Mapping the literature of transcultural nursing. J Med Libr Assoc 2005;94:143–51.
4. Leininger M. Transcultural nursing: the study and practice field. Imprint 1991;38: 55–66.

5. Leininger M. Reflections on Nightingale with a focus on human care theory and leadership. Commemorative edition. In: Carroll DP, editor. Notes on nursing. Philadelphia: J.B. Lippincott; 1992. p. 28–38.
6. Carnegie Endowment for International Peace. What is globalization. Available at: http://www.globalization101.org/What_is_Globalization.html. Accessed May 19, 2009.
7. Buerhaus PI, Staiger DO, Auerbach DI. The future of the nursing workforce in the United States: data, trends and implications. Sudbury (MA): Jones and Bartlett Publishers; 2008.
8. US Department of Health and Human Services. 2000. The registered nurse population: findings from the national sample survey. Available at: ftp://ftp.hrsa.gov/bhpr/rnsurvey2000/rnsurvey00.pdf. Accessed May 19, 2009.
9. US Census Bureau. Census 2000 data for the United States. In United States census 2000. Available at: http://www.census.gov/census2000/states/us.html. 2003;. Accessed May 19, 2009.
10. US Department of Health and Human Services. The registered nurse population: findings from the 2004 national sample. Available at: http://bhpr.hrsa.gov/healthworkforce/rnsurvey04/appendixa.htm. Accessed June 25, 2007.
11. Buerhaus PI, Saiger DO, Auerbach DI. Why are shortages of hospital RNs concentrated in specialty care units? Nurs Econ 2000;18:111–6.
12. Cordonez JA. Recruitment, retention and management of generation X: a focus on nursing professionals. J Healthc Manag 2002;47:237–49.
13. Kupperschmidt BR. Understanding generation X employees. J Nurs Adm 1998; 28:3–43.
14. "The Florence Nightingale Pledge." Available at: http://www.nursingworld.org/FunctionalMenuCategories/AboutANA/WhereWeComeFrom_1/FlorenceNightingalePledge.aspx. Accessed June 7, 2009.
15. American Nurses Association. Guide to the code of ethics for nurses. Washington, DC: American Nurses Publishing; 2008.
16. Fowler M. A chronicle of the evolution of the code for nurses. In: White GB, editor. Ethical dilemmas in contemporary nursing practice. Washington, DC: American Nurses Publishing; 2001. p. 149–54.
17. American Nurses Association. Code of ethics for nurses with interpretive statements. Washington, DC: American Nurses Publishing; 2001.
18. American Nurses Association. Cultural diversity in nursing practice. Available at: http://nursingworld.org/readroom/position/ethicsetcldv.htm. Accessed March 19, 2006.
19. American Nurses Association. Nursing's social policy statement. Washington, DC: American Nurses Publishing; 2003.
20. American Nurses Association. Nursing scope and standards of practice. Washington, DC: American Nurses Publishing; 2004.
21. Stokes L. Ten ways to operationalize your diversity process Available at: www.prisminternational.com. Accessed May 8, 2009.
22. Burke RJ, Ng E. The changing nature of work and organizations: implications for human resource management. Hum Resource Manag Rev 2006;16:86–94.
23. Heller BR, Oros MT, Durney-Crowley J. The future of nursing education: ten trends to watch. Available at: http://www.nln.org/nlnjournal/infotrends.htm. Accessed May 8, 2009.
24. Crawford C, Harrington C, Estes CL. Health policy: crisis and reform in the U.S. health care delivery system. San Francisco: Jossey-Bass; 2004.
25. Hopkins WE, Sterkel-Powell K, Hopkins SA. Training priorities for a diverse work force. Public Pers Manage 1994;23:429–36.

26. Fine MG. Cultural diversity in the workplace: the state of the field. J Bus Com 1996;33:485–502.
27. Seymen OA. The cultural diversity phenomenon in organizations and different approaches for effective cultural diversity management: a literary review. Int J Cross Cult Manag 2006;13:296–315.
28. Swanson JW. Diversity: creating an environment of inclusiveness. Nurs Adm Q 2004;28:207–11.
29. Leininger M. Founder's focus: transcultural nursing is discovery of self and the world of others. J Transcult Nurs 2000;11:312–3.
30. Marriner-Tomey A. Guide to nursing management and leadership. 8th edition. St. Louis (MO): Mosby Elsevier; 2009.
31. Betancourt JR, Green AR, Carrillo JE. Cultural competence in health care: emerging frameworks and practical approaches. New York: Commonwealth Fund, Quality of Care for Underserved Populations; 2002. Available at: http://www.cmwf.org/usr_doc/betancourt_culturalcompetence_576.pdf. Accessed June 7, 2009.
32. Georgetown University Center for Child and Human Development, National Center for Cultural Competence. Cultural competence health practitioner assessment. Available at: http://www11.georgetown.edu/research/gucchd/nccc/foundations/need.html. Accessed May 3, 2009.
33. American College of Healthcare Executives, the American Hospital Association, the National Center for Leadership, and the Institute for Diversity in Health Management. Strategies for leadership: does your hospital reflect the community it serves?. Available at: www.aha.org/aha/key_issues/disparity/content/DiversityTool.pdf. Accessed May 3, 2009.
34. Kripalani S, Weiss B. Teaching about health literacy and clear communication. J Gen Intern Med 2006;21:888–90.
35. Institute of Medicine. In the nation's compelling interest: ensuring diversity in the health care workforce. Washington, DC: National Academy Press; 2004.
36. Cohen JJ, Gabriel BA, Terrell C. The case for diversity in the health care workforce. Health Aff 2002;21:90–102.
37. US Department of Health and Human Services. The rationale for diversity in the health professions: a review of the evidence. Available at: ftp://ftp.hrsa.gov/bhpr/workforce/diversity.pdf. Accessed May 8, 2009.

# From Means to Ends: Artificial Nutrition and Hydration

Cheryl Monturo, PhD, MBE, CRNP[a], Kevin Hook, MA, MSN, CRNP[b],*

KEYWORDS

- Ethics • Artificial nutrition • Hydration
- Decision-making • Reasoning

The withdrawal, withholding, or implementation of life-sustaining treatments such as artificial nutrition and hydration challenge nurses on a daily basis. To meet these challenges, nurses need the composite skills of moral and ethical discernment, practical wisdom and a knowledge base that justifies reasoning and actions that support patient and family decision making. Nurses' moral knowledge develops through experiential learning, didactic learning, and deliberation of ethical principles that merge with moral intuition, ethical codes, and moral theories. Only when a nurse becomes skilled and confident in gathering empiric and ethical knowledge can he or she fully act as a moral agent in assisting families faced with making highly emotional decisions regarding the provision, withholding, or withdrawal of artificial nutrition and hydration.

## NURSING KNOWLEDGE

There are ways of "knowing" that underpin how nurses reason and act concerning the use and effectiveness of artificial nutrition and hydration (ANH). Among these reasons are those that nurse theorist Barbara Carper suggested in her seminal work published in 1978 entitled "Fundamental Ways of Knowing in Nursing," in which she suggests a typology of nursing knowledge using 4 patterns: empirics, ethics, personal, and esthetic.[1] Two of these patterns are particularly relevant and support the notion that moral reasoning and action cannot occur in the absence of empiric knowledge combined with ethics education. These ways of knowing are implicated in the daily decisions that challenge nurses regarding ANH.

### Empiric Knowledge

Empiric knowledge represents the science of nursing, providing verifiable factual and descriptive information that can be applied to a clinical situation. ANH is the delivery of

[a] West Chester University College of Health Sciences, Department of Nursing, 222C Sturzebecker Health Sciences Center, West Chester, PA 19383, USA
[b] Advanced Practice Nursing and Ethics Integration, Golden Living Living Centers, 7 MacArthur Boulevard, #1607, Westmont, NJ 08108, USA
* Corresponding author.
E-mail address: kevin.hook@goldenliving.com (K. Hook).

Nurs Clin N Am 44 (2009) 505–515
doi:10.1016/j.cnur.2009.07.005
0029-6465/09/$ – see front matter © 2009 Elsevier Inc. All rights reserved.

nursing.theclinics.com

nutrients via the gastrointestinal tract, the vascular system, or subcutaneously for hydration alone. This life-sustaining treatment nourishes patients in varying degrees and with greater or lesser success in a variety of clinical states, including persistent vegetative state (PVS), advanced progressive dementia, and other terminal illnesses, and in several temporary or chronic conditions. ANH in the form of enteral nutrition is commonly administered through the gastrointestinal tract either through a temporary or permanent enteral tube. According to reports from the *National Hospital Discharge Survey,* approximately 279 000 permanent enteral tubes were placed in 2005,[2] a 3-fold increase over the past 20 years.[3] Some of this increase may be attributed to improved technology in the development of the percutaneous endoscopic gastrostomy in 1980, which requires no major surgery or general anesthesia.[4]

ANH is an effective and viable therapy for temporary or chronic conditions that affect the ingestion of food and fluids. Some literature demonstrates that ANH prolongs life, improves survival and nutritional status, and improves quality of life in limited instances. Such situations include nourishment for individuals with a temporary inability to use the gastrointestinal tract because of a nonterminal illness or the need for a time trial to examine a patient's chance for recovery. In those instances, ANH is clearly not only physiologically useful but qualitatively beneficial.[5,6] Its advantage in many other clinical settings is questionable and may reflect knowledge differences about the goals of care.[7]

For patients in a terminal state or others who are severely ill, there is large body of evidence regarding ANH's lack of efficacy to prolong life or reduce symptom burden. Evidence is conflicting or fails to show that ANH affects the survival rate of severely ill patients,[8] patients receiving chemotherapy,[7,9–11] or the complication rates after cancer surgery.[12–14] Results are also mixed when examining the literature on hydration alone. Hydration of terminally ill patients resulted in poorer nutritional status and the lack of a strong association between clinical signs of dehydration and fluid balance.[15] This finding compares to a more positive outcome from hydration of cancer patients, in which they describe a lower symptom burden.[16] Unlike these conflicting reports, a significant body of knowledge seems to support a lack of evidence to show improved survival in patients with dementia.[17–22]

Support for ANH use in other disease states is mixed. In postoperative patients with upper gastrointestinal neoplasms and patients receiving radiation therapy for advanced head and neck cancers, ANH was shown to decrease morbidity and improve nutritional status.[12,23,24] ANH also may prolong life in patients with bulbar amyotrophic lateral sclerosis,[25,26] acute stroke with dysphagia or head injury,[27,28] short-term critical care status,[29] and extreme short-bowel syndrome.[30] PVS poses special considerations for many, but there is little evidence to support that ANH contributes to an improvement in quality of life.[31] The physiologic response of persons in vegetative states to ANH may differ from those who are actively dying and may not appear as burdensome. The lack of a clear pathology in PVS further compounds the issue.[32] ANH may prolong life in PVS, leaving patients in this state of unawareness for years.[31,33] Given the inconsistent evidence concerning the impact of ANH, some might assume that it may be helpful but cannot be harmful. Despite this assumption, most nurses are well aware of the considerable risks associated with ANH, including aspiration pneumonia, diarrhea, catheter and tube site infections, mobility limitations during infusion, and self-extubation.[19,34–36]

Finally, clarification of empiric knowledge related to the effect of the absence of nutrition, hydration, or both treatments simultaneously is necessary. Unfortunately, there is little evidence to support or refute the presence or lack of distressing symptoms as a result of removal of ANH or hydration. Physiologically, starvation can be described as the "depletion of food stores in the body tissues."[37] The main effect of starvation is the depletion of protein and fat stores caused by limited carbohydrate stores in the body; patients eventually succumb to a loss of body protein.[38] Symptomatically, patients exhibit the primary result of acidosis—central nervous system depression manifested by disorientation and eventual coma.[37] In addition to acidosis, some postulate that starvation may be accompanied by an increase in endorphin release, thereby creating a sense of elation,[39] which some believe is the basis for claims of analgesia or anesthesia in terminally ill patients who refuse food.[40]

Data regarding symptoms that result from dehydration are controversial. Some argue that this phenomenon is painless and not distressing,[20,41,42] whereas others found that dehydration resulted in thirst, agitated delirium, neuromuscular irritability, and nausea.[43–46] The experience of caregivers supports the notion that dehydration is an acceptable and comfortable manner in which to die.[47] Evidence suggests a connection between the more experienced caregiver and a higher level of acceptance.[48] Despite the findings of "The President's Commission for the Study of Ethical Problems in Medicine and Biomedical and Behavioral Research"[49] in 1983, which found no moral or ethical distinction between artificial nutrition and other life-sustaining treatments, there seems to be a societal disconnect in categorizing ANH as either a life-sustaining treatment or a basic ordinary need. It is also possible that ANH may be classified as a medical intervention in patients with a terminal illness but as basic nursing or ancillary care in patients with chronic nonfatal conditions.[33]

## Ethical Knowledge

Carper writes that ethical knowing examines the intersection between knowledge and reasoning, which ultimately directs action in terms of nurses' duties, obligations, and moral imperatives.[1] Professional ethics codes, then, can serve as the end result and the framework for ethical knowledge and ethical reflection.

### Ethical codes

Knowledge of ANH treatment, benefits, and burdens provides a basis for application of ethics and morality. In general, the term "ethics" is used broadly to define the evaluation and understanding of the moral life.[50] Concomitantly, morality addresses social norms concerning personal conduct: right versus wrong, behaviors, character, and motives.[50] For professionals, guideposts for morality in health care are codified through ethical codes. In nursing, the beginning stages of an ethical code date to more than a century ago.[51] This was followed by development of the International Council of Nurses (ICN) code of ethics in the mid-1950s.[52] Although different in specific focus, these codes reflect the same basic principles highlighting the profession's expected standards of behavior and conduct.

The "Code of Ethics for Nurses with Interpretive Statements"[53] does not specifically address ANH or any other particular life-sustaining therapies. It does, however, use a variety of ethical theories and addresses the 4 basic principles in biomedical ethics (autonomy, beneficence, nonmaleficence, and justice) to assist nurses in deliberating ethical dilemmas and outlining broad ethical postures.[53]

### Ethical theories and principles

In any discussion of ethics, it is useful to refer to philosophy and standard theories of morality that provide a basis for moral reasoning and action. According to renowned philosophers Tom Beauchamp and James Childress,[50] ethics describes how society understands and examines the moral life in terms of decision making. Nurses may develop an awareness of an evolving ethical conflict that may be characterized by the dichotomy of following orders for order's sake or creating good for most patients. Following orders is an example of a deontologic perspective. This theory focuses on duties. A proponent of deontologic ethics views moral action as one in which the moral agent (the nurse) acts based on perception of duty, de-emphasizing individual feelings and societal consequences.[54] Correct actions then come from a sense of knowing what is right and not to avoid or promote other consequences. In other words, morality and doing "good" are not predicated on producing happiness or other perceived positive consequences but are intrinsically valuable.[55]

Utilitarianism, in contrast, is the ethical theory of utility. Goodness is equated with happiness or pleasure with a goal of providing the most good for the greatest number of individuals. Right and wrong acts are evaluated based on whether they cause happiness. Unlike deontology, utilitarianism accepts the adage that the end may justify the means.[54,56]

Although comprehensive ethical theories provide an underpinning for decision making, additional knowledge in the form of the 4 basic principles is necessary. In Western medical ethics, these principles have historically informed ethical discussions and include autonomy, beneficence, nonmaleficence, and justice. Autonomy is self-rule that is free from both controlling interference by others and inadequate understanding that prevents meaningful choice. Consequently, it is the basis of informed consent. Respect for patients flows from the principle of autonomy. Discussions and concerns about patient competence are informed by this principle of respect for autonomy.

The principle of autonomy was codified with the passage of the Patient Self-Determination Act (PSDA) in 1990. The PSDA requires health care institutions that receive federal funding in the form of Medicare or Medicaid payments to ask patients if they have or would like to complete an advance directive. The advance directive provides patients with the opportunity to make their health care wishes known when they no longer are able to effectively communicate these wishes to health care providers. Despite the well-intentioned nature of this legislation and the use of advance directives, some feel this has been less than successful in promoting the autonomy of patients and has proven to fail frequently.[57,58]

Beneficence is a moral obligation to act for the benefit of others and implies acts of mercy, kindness, and charity. Some acts of beneficence are obligatory and some are not. Although one is always required never to do harm, one is not always required to do good. Relationships, either personal or professional, require different responsibilities in performing acts of beneficence. Utilitarianism is based on beneficence. It includes protecting the rights of others, preventing harm from occurring to others, removing conditions that cause harm to others, and rescuing persons in danger.[59]

The principle of nonmaleficence is the obligation not to inflict harm on others. Broadly, it means not depriving others of the goods of life. More specifically, rules that emanate from this principle focus on avoiding the infliction of pain or suffering on others.[59] Although beneficence and nonmaleficence may seem like two sides of a coin, obligations not to harm others are frequently more stringent than obligations to help them.[59] The principle of justice includes notions of fairness and equality for all and may be applied to health care situations in terms of fair distribution of resources, whether scarce or plentiful. This is potentially important to the nurse when organizational ethics conflict with the care of an individual.

## REASONING

Reason defined as a "statement offered in explanation or justification" is "the power of comprehending, inferring, or thinking, especially in orderly rational ways."[60]

Reasoning may be seen in this context as the exercise of decision making. Up to this point, the nurse has gathered empiric knowledge in the form of scientific evidence and applied moral knowledge from professional codes of ethics, ethical theories, and principles. Dealing with value differences that result in ethical dilemmas involving the use, withdrawal, or withholding of ANH may be examined within the framework of the previously described ethical theories and principles. Classification of ANH as a medical treatment or basic care and the degree to which burdens or benefits of this treatment are addressed frequently frame the discussion of this intervention.

Ethically, no distinction is made between ANH and other life-sustaining treatments,[49] and there is no moral difference between the withdrawal of ANH and the withholding of ANH.[59,61] Despite this, many practitioners report feeling a visceral difference in withdrawing treatment because it is more "active" and seems to be the sole cause of the patient's eventual demise. Some states have placed different or higher standards on the withdrawal of ANH, further complicating this issue for many nurses.[62] Ideally, nurses can reason through the dilemmas associated with the provision, withholding, or withdrawal of ANH by using an ethical decision-making process. Although there are many models for decision making, most include 4 steps similar to the nursing process. Bosek and Savage include the following 4 actions: (1) identify the ethical problem, (2) identify and consider alternatives, (3) implement a choice, and (4) evaluate the decision-making process and its outcome.[56] Nurses' lack of confidence and knowledge of this process and the ethical components at work can create confusion and uncertainty resulting in exacerbation of already established ethical dilemmas.[63]

Evidence suggests that nursing students analyze ethical dilemmas from a personal moral posture, whereas experienced nurses eventually acquiesce to institutional goals and ethical frameworks, which may be at odds with professional and personal ethics. Consequently, continuing education is necessary for nurses to participate meaningfully as moral agents.[63] Evaluating nursing students' responses to ethical vignettes in the clinical setting at the beginning of nursing education and then at the end of a 4-year program, Nolan and Marker[64] found that nursing students did not consider their clinical experiences as influential in their ethical development as much as ethics coursework. This finding further supports the argument that nurses require increased exposure to ethics education. The lack of sound reasoning may be attributed to the lack of empiric and ethical knowledge consequently impeding a rational and orderly process in ethical decision making.

Because of the pace which with nurses are required to work, ethical education training and the development of sound ethical reasoning and beliefs are worth the effort. Engaging in activities that create time and space for serious ethical deliberation can help create effective ethical decision making when there is no time to engage in lengthy discourse. In this way, the practice of sound ethical analysis may become routine. Allmark[65] suggested that excellence in practice is based on the development of good habits.

In nursing education, evidence indicates that ethical development and the ability to discern ethical dilemmas rely more on deciding that behaviors or actions are "right" rather than on being able to analyze an issue.[66] The ability to think critically about an ethical argument is necessary and is about more than providing a solution to a problem. Exemplifying practical wisdom, ethical judgments need to be supported by good reasons, the absence of which renders any ethical analysis weak. As clinical knowledge increases, the nurse is able to understand how theory can inform practice. Dreyfus and Dreyfus[67] agreed and observed that beginner nurses follow rules but expert nurses trust intuition, knowing that nursing is a place where "theory and practice intertwine in a mutually supportive bootstrapping process as a nurse develop(s) his or her skill." They conclude that both need to be cultivated.[68]

Not uncommonly, when end-of-life decisions are being made, nurses experience moral distress, which is defined as "pain or suffering affecting the body, a bodily part, or the mind."[69] The experience of "moral distress" is explained as a result of nurses having to live with another's decision versus being the one who is the decision-maker, hence distress. An increased sense of moral agency through formal ethics education assists nurses in ameliorating these effects and allows a more open dialogue.[70]

### The Symbolism of Food

Adding to the ANH dilemma, some assume that ANH and food are synonymous and, as such, find the issue of withdrawal or withholding of this life-sustaining treatment a difficult and highly emotional topic. The meaning of food is thoroughly discussed in anthropologic and sociologic literature in terms of the social, religious, and personal significance for behaviors attributed to food and eating.[71] In particular, personal meanings of food are based on social and emotional needs,[72–74] especially those experienced early in life.[75] In this context, food represents a social norm and a significant symbol of life.[73,74,76,77] The imbalance of literature between anthropology, sociology, and health care on this topic may account for the continued confusion as to the placement of ANH into life-sustaining treatments or symbolic and basic care.[78] Nurses must reason through personal, professional, and institutional values, acknowledging the reality of this emotive issue.

### TO ACT

Nurses act in different ways based on their level of experience and variety of clinical exposures. Noting the novice-to-expert theory, Benner[68] described nursing as a clinical practice in which theory becomes relevant as nurses progress along the continuum. Assuming this process may be applied to the development of ethical skill and sensitivity, it is plausible to suggest that nurses with basic knowledge of ethical theories and principles are at the beginning of the continuum. This knowledge, along with continued ethics education, may only be evident and useful as nurses mature in their professional life. Others argue that development of clinical skills is different from ethical skills in that nurses arrive at undergraduate education already equipped with a moral sense.[67] At issue, then, is whether this moral sense is a personal one with roots in a particular religious or cultural background and requires further professional maturation.

Using the decision-making process, the nurse reasons through all aspects of the ANH dilemma and arrives at a conclusion that is intellectually and internally consistent, morally sound, and provides a rationale for the intended actions. Through this process the nurse addresses the conflicts among caregivers, family, and patients as to whether ANH is an appropriate treatment for a patient. Evidence suggests that ethics education has a positive influence on moral action in nurses.[79] The combination of personal moral postures and basic and continuing ethics education provides a foundation for professional maturation. As a result, nurses may develop increased clinical understanding that creates new possibilities for moral agency, defined as the ability to act.[68,80] The degree to which nurses understand and subsequently act on their own moral agency is determined by the depth and skill of their ethical analysis. A strong sense of moral agency, supported by ethics education, is vital to the nurse's ability to act confidently.

## SUMMARY

To achieve meaningful ends to the controversies that arise in the provision of ANH, various measures have been used. Each measure entails requisite skills of knowing, justifying, and acting with empiric and ethical perspectives. Given the preponderance of controversial issues associated with the provision, withholding, and withdrawal of ANH, there is an obligation to strike a balance between those who may benefit and those who do not. This balance should be based on scientific evidence as to the burdens and benefits of ANH.[7,81] This risk/benefit analysis includes the need for expert clinical and ethical skills as ANH and its inherent symbolic meanings evoke highly emotional responses.

Nurses' obligations also require a clear understanding of the foundational ethical principles of autonomy, beneficence, justice, and nonmaleficence. Knowledge of ethical theories helps nurses justify their ethical stance. Understanding the empiric evidence related to the benefits and burdens of ANH helps nurses serve patients and families when offering clinical advice and mediating ethical discussions. Decisions regarding the appropriate use of ANH necessitate the interplay of empiric knowledge, personal moral sense, and application of ethical theories and principles and are the means by which nurses support those ends important to patients and families.

## REFERENCES

1. Carper BA. Fundamental patterns of knowing in nursing. ANS Adv Nurs Sci 1978; 1(1):13–23.
2. De Frances CJ, Cullen KA, Kozak LJ. National hospital discharge survey: 2005 annual summary with detailed diagnoses and procedure data. National Center for Health Statistics 2007;Vital Health Stat 13(165).
3. Graves EJ. Detailed diagnoses and procedures, national hospital discharge survey, 1988. National Center for Health Statistics 1991;Vital Health Stat 13(107).
4. Ponsky JL, Gauderer MW. Percutaneous endoscopic gastrostomy: a nonoperative technique for feeding gastrostomy. Gastrointest Endosc 1981;27(1):9–11.
5. Fine RL. Ethical issues in artificial nutrition and hydration. Nutr Clin Pract 2006;21: 118–25.
6. Goodhall L. Tube feeding dilemmas: can artificial nutrition and hydration be legally or ethically withheld or withdrawn? J Adv Nurs 1997;25:217–22.
7. Suter P, Rogers J, Strack C. Artificial nutrition and hydration for the terminally ill: a reasoned approach. Home Healthc Nurse 2008;26(1):23–9.
8. Rabeneck L, Wray NP, Petersen NJ. Long-term outcomes of patients receiving percutaneous endoscopic gastrostomy tubes. J Gen Intern Med 1996;11(5): 287–93.
9. Yamada N, Koyama H, Hioki K, et al. Effect of postoperative total parenteral nutrition (TPN) as an adjunct to gastrectomy for advanced gastric carcinoma. Br J Surg 1983;70:267–74.
10. Shamberger RC, Brennan MF, Goodgame JT Jr, et al. A prospective, randomized study of adjuvant parenteral nutrition in the treatment of sarcomas: results of metabolic and survival studies. Surgery 1984;96:1–13.
11. Popp MB, Fisher RI, Wesley R, et al. A prospective randomized study of adjuvant parenteral nutrition in the treatment of advanced diffuse lymphoma: influence on survival. Surgery 1981;90:195–203.
12. Daly JM, Hearne B, Dunaj J, et al. Nutritional rehabilitation in patients with advanced head and neck cancer receiving radiation therapy. Am J Surg 1984; 148(4):514–20.

13. Daly JM, Weintraub FN, Shou J, et al. Enteral nutrition during multimodality therapy in upper gastrointestinal cancer patients. Ann Surg 1995;221:327–38.

14. Brennan MF, Pisters PW, Posner M, et al. A prospective randomized trial of total parenteral nutrition after major pancreatic resection for malignancy. Ann Surg 1994;220:436–41.

15. Morita T, Hyodo I, Yaoshimi T, et al. Artificial hydration therapy, laboratory findings, and fluid balance in terminally ill patients with abdominal malignancies. J Pain Symptom Manage 2005;31(2):130–9.

16. Bruera E, Sala R, Rico MR, et al. Effects of parenteral hydration in terminally ill cancer patients: a preliminary study. J Clin Oncol 2005;23(10):2366–71.

17. Sanders DS, Anderson AJ, Bardham KD. Percutaneous endoscopic gastrostomy: an effective strategy for gastrostomy feeding in patients with dementia. Clin Med 2004;4:235–41.

18. Gillick MR. Rethinking the role of tube feeding in patients with advanced dementia [see comment]. N Engl J Med 2000;342(3):206–10.

19. Finucane TE, Christmas C, Travis K. Tube feeding in patients with advanced dementia: a review of the evidence [comment]. J Am Med Assoc 1999; 282(14):1365–70.

20. Post SG. Tube feeding and advanced progressive dementia. Hastings Cent Rep 2001;31(1):36–42.

21. Mitchell SL, Kiely DK, Lipsitz LA. Does artificial enteral nutrition prolong the survival of institutionalized elders with chewing and swallowing problems? J Gerontol A Biol Sci Med Sci 1998;53:M207–13.

22. Meier DE, Ahronheim JC, Morris J, et al. High short-term mortality in hospitalized patients with advanced dementia: lack of benefit of tube feeding. Arch Intern Med 2001;161:594–9.

23. Lee JH, Macktay M, Unger LD. Prophylactic gastrostomy tubes in patients undergoing intensive irradiation for cancer of the head and neck. Arch Otolaryngol Head Neck Surg 1998;124:871–5.

24. Senkal M, Zumtobel V, Bauer KH, et al. Outcome and cost effectiveness of perioperative enteral immunonutrition in patients undergoing elective upper gastrointestinal tract surgery: a prospective randomized study. Arch Surg 1999;134:1309–16.

25. Mazzini L, Corra T, Zaccala M, et al. Percutaneous endoscopic gastrostomy and enteral nutrition in amyotrophic lateral sclerosis. J Neurol 1995;242:695–8.

26. Miller RG. Examining the evidence about treatment in ALS/MND. Amyotroph Lateral Scler Other Motor Neuron Disord 2001;2:3–7.

27. Rapp RP, Young B, Twyman D, et al. The favorable effect of early parenteral feeding on survival in head-injured patients. J Neurosurg 1983;58:906–12.

28. Wanklyn P, Cox N, Belfield P. Outcome in patients who require a gastrostomy after stroke. Age Ageing 1995;24:510–4.

29. Martin CM, Doig GS, Heyland DK, et al. Multicentre, cluster-randomized clinical trial of algorithms for critical-care enteral and parenteral therapy (ACCEPT). Can Med Assoc J 2004;170:197–204.

30. Scolapio JS, Fleming CR, Kelly D, et al. Survival of home parenteral nutrition-treated patients: 20 years of experience at the Mayo Clinic. Mayo Clin Proc 1999;74:217–22.

31. Ganzini L. Artificial nutrition at the end of life: ethics and evidence. Palliat Support Care 2006;4:135–43.

32. Schiff ND, Ribary U, Rodriquez Moreno D, et al. Residual cerebral activity and behavioural fragments can remain in the persistently vegetative brain. Brain 2002; 125:1210–34.

33. Gigli GL, Valente M. The withdrawal of nutrition and hydration in the vegetative state patient: societal dimension and issues at stake for the medical profession. NeuroRehabilitation 2004;19:315–28.
34. Fuhrman MP, Herrmann VM. Bridging the continuum: nutrition support in palliative and hospice care. Nutr Clin Pract 2006;21:134–41.
35. Ciocon JO, Silverstone FA, Graver LM, et al. Tube feedings in elderly patients: indications, benefits, and complications. Arch Intern Med 1988;148(2):429–33.
36. Callahan CM, Haag KM, Weinberger M, et al. Outcomes of percutaneous endoscopic gastrostomy among older adults in a community setting [comment]. J Am Geriatr Soc 2000;48(9):1048–54.
37. Guyton AC, Hall JE. Textbook of medical physiology. 10th edition. Philadelphia: WB Saunders; 2000. p. 809.
38. Saudek CD, Felig P. The metabolic events of starvation. Am J Med 1976;60: 117–26.
39. Cohen BJ. Theory and practice of psychiatry. New York: Oxford University Press; 2003.
40. Meares CJ. Primary caregivers perceptions of intake cessation in patients who are terminally ill. Oncol Nurs Forum 1997;24:1751–7.
41. Hoefler J. Making decisions about tube feeding for severely demented patients at the end of life: clinical, legal, and ethical considerations. Death Stud 2000;24: 233–54.
42. Billings JA. Comfort measures for the terminally ill: is dehydration painful? J Am Geriatr Soc 1985;33:808–10.
43. Sutcliffe J. Palliative care: terminal dehydration. Nurs Times 1994;90:60–3.
44. Morita T, Tei Y, Tsunoda J, et al. Determinants of the sensation of thirst in terminally ill cancer patients. Support Care Cancer 2001;9(3):177–86.
45. Lawlor PG, Gagnon B, Mancini IL, et al. Occurrence, causes and outcome of delirium in patients with advanced cancer: a prospective study. Arch Intern Med 2000;160:786–94.
46. Fainsinger RL, Bruera E. When to treat dehydration in a terminally ill patient? Support Care Cancer 1997;5(3):205–11.
47. Andrews M, Levine A. Dehydration in the terminal patient: perception of hospice nurses. Am J Hosp Care 1989;6(1):31–4.
48. Luchins DJ, Hanrahan P. What is appropriate healthcare for end stage dementia? J Am Geriatr Soc 1993;41:25–30.
49. The President's Commission for the Study of Ethical Problems in Medicine and Biomedical and Behavioral Research. Deciding to forego life-sustaining treatment. Washington, DC: US Government Printing Office; 1983.
50. Beauchamp TL, Childress JF. Principles of biomedical ethics. 5th edition. New York: Oxford University Press; 2001.
51. American Nurses Association. Code of ethics for nurses with interpretive statements. Washington, DC: American Nurses Publishing; 2001. Available at: http://nursingworld.org/ethics/code/protected_nwcoe813.htm.
52. International Council of Nurses. The ICN code of ethics for nurses. Geneva, Switzerland: ICN; 2000. Available at: http://www.icn.ch/icncode.pdf.
53. American Nurses Association. Code of ethics for nurses with interpretative statements. Silver Spring (MD): American Nurses Association; 2001.
54. Dahnke M, Dreher HM. Defining ethics and applying the theories. In: Lachman V, editor. Applied ethics in nursing. New York: Springer Publishing; 2006. p. 3–13.
55. Pojman L. Who are we: theories of human nature. New York: Oxford University Press; 2006.

56. DeWolf Bosek MS, Savage TA. The ethical component of nursing education: integrating ethics into clinical experience. Philadelphia: Lippincott Williams and Wilkins; 2007.
57. Ulrich L. The patient self-determination act: meeting the challenges in patient care. Washington, DC: Georgetown University Press; 1999.
58. Fagerlin A, Schneider CE. Enough: the failure of the living will. Hastings Cent Rep 2004;34(2):30–42.
59. Beauchamp TL, Childress JF. Principles of biomedical ethics. 6th edition. New York: Oxford University Press; 2008.
60. Merriam Webster. Definition reason. Available at: http://www.merriam-webster.com/dictionary/reason. Accessed February 24, 2009.
61. Jonson R, Siegler M, Winslade W. Clinical ethics: a practical approach to ethical decisions in clinical medicine. 6th Edition. New York: Lippincott Williams & Wilkins; 2006.
62. Seiger CE, Arnold JF, Ahronheim JC. Refusing artificial nutrition and hydration: does statutory law send the wrong message? J Am Geriatr Soc 2002;50:544–50.
63. Ham K. Principled thinking: a comparison of nursing students and experienced nurses. J Contin Educ Nurs 2004;35(2):66–73.
64. Nolan P, Market D. Ethical reasoning observed: a longitudinal study of nursing students. Nurs Ethics 2002;9(3):243–58.
65. Allmark P. Can the study of ethics enhance nursing practice? J Adv Nurs 2004; 51(6):618–24.
66. Holt J, Long T. Moral guidance, moral philosophy, and moral issues in practice. Nurse Educ Today 1999;19:246–9.
67. Dreyfus H, Dreyfus S. The relationship of theory and practice in the acquisition of skills. In: Benner P, Tanner C, Chesla C, editors. Expertise in nursing practice: caring, clinical judgment and ethics. New York: Springer Publishing; 1996. p. 29–47.
68. Benner P, Tanner C, Chesla C. Expertise in nursing practice: caring, clinical judgment and ethics. New York: Springer Publishing; 1996.
69. Webster Merriam. Definition moral distress. Available at: http://www.merriam-webster.com/dictionary/distress. Accessed March 9, 2009.
70. Oberle K, Hughes D. Doctors' and nurses' perceptions of ethical problems in end-of-life decision. J Adv Nurs 2001;33(6):707–15.
71. Monturo CA. A cultural exploration of aging veterans: the meaning of food and beliefs regarding artificial nutrition at end-of-life [dissertation]. Philadelphia: School of Nursing, University of Pennsylvania; 2005.
72. Arnold C. Nutrition intervention in the terminally ill cancer patient. J Am Diet Assoc 1986;86(4):522–3.
73. Caspar R. Food and water: symbol and reality. Health Prog 1988;69(4):54–8.
74. Schmitz P. The process of dying with and without feeding and fluids by tube. Law Med Health Care 1991;19(1/2):23–6.
75. Fieldhouse P. Food and nutrition: customs and culture. Dover (NH): Croom Helm; 1986.
76. Lynn T, Childress SF. Must patients always be given food and water? Hastings Cent Rep 1983;13:17–21.
77. McInerney F. Provision of food and fluids in terminal care: a sociological analysis. Soc Sci Med 1992;34(11):1271–6.
78. Monturo CA. The meaning of food: a cultural model of community identity and social memory in aging veterans at end-of-life. Accepted Journal of Clinical Nursing.

79. Grady C, Danis M, Soeken KL, et al. Does ethics education influence the moral action of practicing nurses and social workers? Am J Bioeth 2008;8(4):4–11.
80. Merriam Webster. Definition agency. Available at: http://www.merriam-webster.com/dictionary/agency. Accessed May 15, 2009.
81. Wagner B, Ersek M, Riddell S. HPNA position statement artificial nutrition and hydration in end-of-life care. 2004. Available at: http://www.hpna.org/pdf/PositionStatement_ArtificialNutritionAndHydration.pdf, Accessed February 24, 2009.

# Nursing, Religiosity, and End-of-Life Care: Interconnections and Implications

Dana Bjarnason, PhD, RN, NE-BC[a,b,]*

KEYWORDS

• End of life • Religiosity • Advocacy
• Religious beliefs • Belief systems

Extraordinary changes in health care in the United States in the late twentieth and early twenty-first centuries have resulted in increasingly difficult challenges relating to the end of life. Unparalleled technological advances, legislative attempts to humanize end-of-life care, and increasing public demands for health care interventions have further complicated an already complex issue. Increasingly mobile populations and the proliferation of approaches to the provision of health care have compounded difficulties by creating impersonal relationships between health care providers and patients. Added to these complexities are unanswered questions about the consequences of the increasing cultural and ethnic diversity of care providers and the recipients of end-of-life care, particularly as it relates to the resultant divergence in religiosity.

## HISTORICAL PERSPECTIVES
### Nursing and End-of-Life Care

Overt controversy about end-of-life care in health care facilities in the United States traces back to 1976 when Karen Ann Quinlan was a patient in a persistent vegetative state whose circumstances were put forward to the New Jersey Supreme Court.[1] Her case was the first in which it was recognized that the implied right to privacy and self-determination of incompetent dying patients could be exercised by surrogates, based on the standard of substituted judgment.[2] A similar case,[3] and the first decision by the US Supreme Court to explicitly recognize the rights of dying patients,[4] spurred Congress to enact the Patient Self-Determination Act of 1990 (PSDA). Among other things, the PSDA required hospitals receiving Medicare funds to implement advance directive policies and to provide education to staff and communities about the PSDA.[5]

---

[a] Ben Taub General Hospital, 1504 Taub Loop, Houston, TX 77030, USA
[b] Quentin Mease Community Hospital, 3601 N MacGregor Way, Houston, TX 77004, USA
* Ben Taub General Hospital, 1504 Taub Loop, Houston, TX 77030.
E-mail address: dana_bjarnason@hchd.tmc.edu

Nurs Clin N Am 44 (2009) 517–525
doi:10.1016/j.cnur.2009.07.010
0029-6465/09/$ – see front matter © 2009 Elsevier Inc. All rights reserved.

It was cases like these, and issues regarding knowledge of the PSDA from the perspective of patients and health care providers, that led to increasing concern among nurses regarding their role in end-of-life discussions.[6-10] Since then, nurses have continued to express concern about their role in the discussion of end-of-life care and decision making.[11-14]

Studies have examined the nurse's role related to care of the patient and, more recently, have focused on the nurse's participation in discussions about decision making and end-of-life care.[12-14] Further complicating end-of-life care issues are appropriate concerns raised by nurses and others about whether end-of-life care accurately reflects the patient's desires and if the consequences of specific choices have been considered by the patient, especially before the implementation of advance directives. Additionally, when patients are unable to make decisions, there are concerns about whether proxy decision makers are appropriate.[15-17]

Recognizing the importance of a consistent and deliberate approach to end-of-life care, the American Nurses Association (ANA) produced a compendium of historic and landmark documents, which was formulated from the questions that nurses were raising. In addition to a directive regarding the management of pain in dying patients, the *Compendium of Position Statements on the Nurse's Role in End-of-Life Decisions*[18] provided nurses with directives that were adopted by the ANA Board of Directors, including *Nursing and the Patient Self-Determination Act, Foregoing Artificial Nutrition and Hydration,* and *Nursing Care and Do-not-Resuscitate Decisions*. Nurses have also added substantially to the end-of-life care dialog and have been instrumental in establishing and participating in programs such as the End-of-Life Nursing Education Consortium[19] and in the nationwide development and implementation of hospice care.[20]

### End-of-Life Care in the United States

In 1995, a landmark study, about a controlled trial to improve care for seriously ill, hospitalized patients, stirred the state of inquiry and research into end-of-life care in the United States. The *Study to Understand Prognoses and Preferences for Outcomes and Risks of Treatment* (SUPPORT) principal investigators identified that there were substantial problems in caring for seriously ill, hospitalized patients. They cited such things as poor communication, overly aggressive treatment, and issues surrounding the death of patients. These issues included lack of knowledge of when patients preferred to avoid CPR (47%), do-not-resuscitate orders that were written within 2 days of death (46%), death of patients after at least 10 days spent in the intensive care unit (38%), and moderate-to-severe pain experienced by 50% of conscious patients who died in the hospital.[17]

In 1997, the Institute of Medicine (IOM) released its first breakthrough document about end-of-life care in the United States. The *Approaching Death: Improving Care at the End of Life* report urged the health care community to build a greater understanding of what constituted good care at the end of life. The report offered specific recommendations to improve end-of-life care, including determining diagnosis and prognosis and communicating them to the patient and family, establishing clinical and personal goals, and matching physical, psychological, spiritual, and practical care strategies to the patient's values and circumstances.[15]

The IOM issued a subsequent report in 2003 entitled *Describing Death in America: What We Need to Know*. The report examined data that was available to track and evaluate the quality of life and care experienced by Americans during the months immediately preceding death. The IOM uncovered wide gaps between what was known and what should be known. The report covered the important tenets of provider accountability for quality care, the projection of future needs, and the importance of the evaluation and improvement of approaches to dying patients. It also called for the advancement of research into clinical, organizational, and financing options for care at the end of life.[16]

Healthcare providers have risen to the challenges, spurred by the publication of the SUPPORT article and the IOM reports. A demonstration project conducted in Alabama provided a comprehensive approach to end-of-life care for safety-net populations. The researchers were able to demonstrate success at changing the location of death for terminally-ill hospital patients from acute care and intensive care units to palliative care settings.[21] Other studies have explored the influence of culture on communication at the end of life.[22,23] A focus group study conducted by Shrank and colleagues[24] found that non-Hispanic white and African American groups differed broadly in the preferred content and structure of end-of-life discussions and on the values that influence those preferences.

One small but intriguing study examined the effects of religiosity on patients' perceptions of do-not-resuscitate (DNR) status.[25] Of the 48 oncology inpatients in the study, 75% said that they understood the meaning of DNR, but only 32% were able to accurately define it.[25] Although certain religious practices, such as meditation and thinking about God, correlated with the belief that DNR decisions were morally wrong, no association was found between religious denomination and the morality of DNR.

Recent studies[25,26] have begun to explore end-of-life care in the national curricula of medical schools and schools of nursing. These studies have found wide support among deans and health care educators for integrating end-of-life education into the curricula.

## RELIGIOSITY DEFINED

Defining religiosity is central to engaging in a discussion about its consequences in relation to patient care and end of life. A recent concept analysis of religiosity found consistent congruity between health care disciplines, including nursing, medicine, and the medical humanities, over many years.[27] Findings revealed considerable consensus relative to the features that characterize religiosity, encompassing three specific foci: (1) association with a religious affiliation (eg, Protestant, Catholic); (2) participating in religious activities (eg, praying, church attendance); and (3) holding religious beliefs (eg, relationship with a higher power, believing in the religious scriptures of their belief, or degree to which religion is important). Therefore, the overarching definition of religiosity, revealed by the analysis, is that religiosity is distinguished by religious affiliation, activities, and beliefs. Furthermore, findings suggest that expressions of religiosity are personal, intrinsic, or internal, (eg, private prayer or reading scriptures) and public, extrinsic, or external (eg, receiving prayer or a religious ritual or participating in religious meetings).[27]

## RELIGIOSITY AND PATIENT CARE

Although the historic ties between health care and religion are well recognized, it has only been in recent years that understanding the importance of religious values and their effect on patient outcomes has received increasing attention in the health care literature.[28–32] More than 25 years ago, Daniel Foster,[33] a distinguished internist and professor of medicine, asserted that there were 4 reasons why physicians must deal with religion in the routine care of patients. He postulated that: (1) religion influences the feelings and actions of a significant number of people, (2) patients often place the physician in the role of secular priest, (3) illness induces serious religious questions, and (4) physicians' own belief systems impinge on and influence patient care. Although these assertions seem straightforward, there has been little research evaluating religiosity from the standpoint of the health care provider.

### Patient Behavior and the Influence of Religion

Foster's first thesis asserts that there is evidence to suggest that patient behavior may be influenced by religion, describing examples wherein care and treatment are enhanced or compromised because of strongly held religious beliefs on the part of the patient or family.[33] Research has shown that high degrees of religiosity have a protective mechanism against suicide,[34] depression,[35] hypertension,[32] and drug involvement.[36] High religiosity has been shown to be associated with improved coping during stressful life events,[29] during times of stress related to illness such as chronic joint pain[28] or depression,[37,38] and during stress associated with psychopathology related to substance use and abuse.[30]

A study explored how physicians interpret and respond when there is conflict between medical recommendations and the patient's religious beliefs.[39] The study found that conflict introduced by religious beliefs was common and occurred in 3 situations: (1) when religious doctrines directly conflict with medical recommendations (eg, the refusal of blood transfusions by Jehovah's Witnesses); (2) when there is controversy within society (eg, end-of-life decisions where conflict arises between the sacredness of life and medically futile treatment); and (3) when there is medical uncertainty and patients choose faith over medicine (eg, "it is in God's hands" or "God will provide").

Conflicts between religiosity and medicine are exemplified by nationally publicized cases wherein parents, based on their religious convictions, have refused to permit interventions such as chemotherapy or blood transfusions for their children.[40] In many of these cases, health care teams and the state become involved because of concerns about religious beliefs endangering a child. These situations illustrate the influence that religion can have on health care and demonstrate the need for nurses to recognize, as Foster emphasizes, that although health care providers are not required, themselves, to believe, they need to know that others believe, sometimes intensely.[33]

### The Nurse as Secular Priest (or Priestess)

Paraphrasing Foster's second thesis, which metaphorically compares the role of the physician to that of a secular priest, is relevant to nursing also.[33] As with religious and medical roles, the role of religion in nursing has been separated professionally. The original version of the Florence Nightingale Pledge required the nurse to pledge before God to pass life in purity and to practice the profession faithfully.[41] This pledge to God is no longer a requirement of nursing's code of ethics.

Changes in society and the role of the professional nurse have greatly diminished the significance of religiosity as a requisite for nursing. However, as the role of the nurse developed significantly in the direction of patient advocacy, the importance of hearing "confession" and providing interpretation for patients has increased. It is common to hear nurses say that patients have failed to report troubling symptoms to the physician, despite having described and discussed concerns during the nursing assessment.

The confessional patient-to-nurse role may also be manifested in other ways. An often-heard example relates to conversations about code status when a physician discusses end-of-life interventions with a terminally ill patient. Patients often request resuscitation, then subsequently query the nurse concerning what resuscitation entails. When informed that the treatment for "starting your heart" consists of cardiac compressions, artificial respiration, defibrillation, and possible intubation that requires transfer to a medical intensive care unit, many patients respond in horror. They "don't want to be on a breathing machine" or they consider themselves "too old and sick" or are concerned about dying without dignity. Clarification often leads to reassessment and to subsequent changes to the goals of patient care.

### Illness and the Serious Questions

Foster's third thesis has profound implications for the study of health care decision making, particularly as it relates to end-of-life care. He states that,

> "it is probably safe to say that most people spend relatively little time contemplating philosophic matters, and certainly not life or death"

and that

> "a presumption of personal immunity is not unusual, even in scholars whose job it is to think, speak, and write about finitude-mortality (philosophers, theologians) or by professionals regularly exposed to death (physicians, nurses, and their colleagues)."[33]

For the most part, these statements ring true, for it is only when our own mortality or the mortality of those who are close to us is in question that we begin seriously, as Foster says, to divert our focus from the ordinary to the extraordinary.

Related to coping strategies, religiosity has been identified and described as the seeking of meaning, purpose, and hope through religion that occurs when patients are confronted with illness or crisis.[38,42,43] Research suggests that black patients rely more heavily on religiosity as a coping strategy. In a study that examined male veterans with moderate to severe chronic hip or knee pain, black subjects were more likely to have tried prayer as a form of therapy and to perceive prayer as helpful in their treatment.[28] Another study showed significant use of religious coping strategies among African Americans with panic disorders.[45]

### The Nurse's Belief and Patient Care

As previously discussed, Foster cautions about problems that may arise when the patient has strong religious beliefs and the doctor has none (or different ones) or, conversely, when the physician is highly religious and the patient is not.[33] This same warning could be applied to the nurse-patient relationship; however, a paucity of literature examines the relationship between nurse religiosity and patient care. Although this is an aspect of care largely missing from the nursing literature, physician researchers have begun to explore the implications of physician religiosity and patient care. One such study looked at the association of physicians' religious characteristics with their attitudes and self-reported behavior patterns regarding religion and spirituality in their encounters with patients. The response rate of 63% (from 2000 surveys mailed to a stratified random sample of practicing physicians) suggests a high degree of interest in the topic. Most physicians in the study (91%) thought that it was appropriate to discuss religious and spirituality issues if the patient desired. Results were more divided on issues of physicians talking about their own religious beliefs or experiences (14% responded that they would never do so, while 43% said only when the patient asks). Fifty-three percent of the sample thought that it was appropriate to pray with patients when they ask, whereas 17% thought that physicians should never pray with their patients. The researchers found that physicians who are more religious and spiritual (particularly Protestants) were significantly more apt to address religion and spirituality with the patient.[44]

Another study conducted with the same sample examined an issue that was recently the focus of media attention—the issue of health professionals who refuse to provide treatment based on moral grounds. This research examined physicians' perceptions of their ethical rights and obligations to patients who request legal medical procedures, for example, terminal sedation in dying patients, abortions for failed contraception, and birth control for adolescents without parental consent. The study results showed a significant association between physicians' judgments about their obligations and their religious characteristics, sex, and beliefs about these controversial medical practices. The study concluded that physicians who were more religious were less likely to offer or provide legal but contentious interventions.[46] In a study conducted to assess beliefs of primary care residents regarding spirituality and religion in clinical encounters, approximately half of the 227 respondents felt that they should take part in their patients' religious or spiritual lives. This feeling was associated with greater frequency of participation by the resident in organized religious activities, higher levels of spirituality, and older resident age.[47]

One last example is a study that explored end-of-life care issues and practices among 443 Jewish physicians working at 4 hospitals in Israel. The researchers found that very religious physicians (as compared with moderately religious or secular physicians) were less likely to believe in withdrawing life-sustaining treatments or to approve the use of pain medication if it would hasten death.[48] There was no significance regarding findings for withholding life-sustaining treatments, although the researchers noted that when caring for a suffering terminally ill patient, very religious physicians were much less likely to stop life-sustaining treatments. The researchers found that there was no relationship between physicians' religiosity and physician-patient communication and that physicians' desire for support in handling issues regarding end-of-life care was universal.[48]

## RELIGIOSITY AND NURSING

Although physicians have begun to explore the more subtle complexities of physician religiosity and its effect on the care of patients, most nursing literature focuses on the importance of being aware of and understanding the patient's spiritual or religious beliefs or needs, rather than on the implications of nurses' religiosity. For example, Musgrave and colleagues[22] explored research data that support a relationship between spirituality and health, particularly among women of color. The investigators concluded that spirituality and religiosity were of significant benefit to the study subjects, having implications for prevention, health-promoting behaviors, and coping with health problems. Wright[49] highlights the professional, ethical, and legal implications for spiritual care in nursing. She cites professional standards, such as the Joint Commission and the International Council of Nurses' Code for Nurses; ethical values, such as fidelity, advocacy, autonomy, and self-determination; and the legal issue of privileged communication to explicate the obligations that nurses have to support the spiritual care of patients.

In an attempt to understand spirituality in the caregiving and care-receiving dynamic, a qualitative study conducted by Theis and colleagues[43] examined spirituality in 60 caregivers and care receivers. Data from the study suggest 2 overarching themes: (1) coping, with subthemes related to formal religion and social support, and (2) meaning, with subthemes of positive attitude, retribution, or reward. The investigators suggest that holistic care could be provided to patients by assessing spirituality, then supporting and enhancing it. Collaboration with clergy and parish nurse programs also was recommended.

Taylor[23] explored the spiritual needs of patients and family caregivers in a study wherein 28 African American and Euro-American patients with cancer and their family caregivers were interviewed. The findings of this study identified similar results for patients and their caregivers, including (1) the needs associated with relating to an Ultimate Other; (2) the need for positivity, hope, and gratitude; (3) the need to give and receive love; (4) the need to review beliefs; (5) the need to have meaning; and (6) the needs related to religiosity and preparation for death. The importance of understanding the manifestation of spiritual needs, and how to talk to patients about these needs, was seen as integral to providing spiritual care to patients. Understanding patient needs was the focus of a tool that Warner[50] developed for spiritual assessment. Created in an attempt to provide nurses with the information to holistically support care provided in emergency situations, the tool presents specific details about beliefs and practices (some relating to end-of-life care) based on religious affiliation.

## SUMMARY

The influence of religious beliefs and practices at the end of life is underinvestigated. Given nursing's advocacy role and the intimate and personal nature of the dimensions of both religiosity and the end of life, exploring the multidimensional interplay of religiosity and end-of-life care is a significant aspect of the nurse-patient relationship and must be better understood. Nurses hold a powerful position in the nurse-patient relationship; therefore, it is vital that nurses understand and respond to the many ways that personal and professional perspectives may influence patient and provider discourse.

A long-held value in nursing relates to supporting the spiritual needs of patients and their families—a need that is exacerbated by the emotional burdens that may accompany the end of life. This spiritual support differs from value-laden subjects, such as the meaning of suffering or end-of-life beliefs, that may be clouded by disparities between the nurse-patient belief systems. To paraphrase Foster, problems arise when the nurse has strong religious beliefs and the patient has none (or different ones) or conversely, when the patient is highly religious and the nurse is not.[33]

The question that must be faced is whether nurses' own belief systems impinge on or influence patient care, especially for patients who are at the end of life. When nurses understand their own beliefs and respect the religious practices and needs of patients and their families, it deepens the humanistic dimensions of the nurse-patient relationship.

## REFERENCES

1. Pence GE. Classic cases about death and dying. 2nd edition. New York: McGraw-Hill, Inc; 1995.
2. In re Quinlan, 70 N.J. 10, 355 A. 2d 647 (1976).
3. In re Conroy, 98 N.J. 321, 364–65, 486 A. 2d 1209 (1985).
4. Cruzan v Director, Missouri Department of Health, 110 S. Ct. 2841 (1990).
5. Patient Self-Determination Act, 42 U.S.C. 1395cc(a) (1990).
6. Hague SB, Moody LE. A study of the public's knowledge regarding advance directives. Nurs Econ 1993;11:303–7.
7. Hassmiller S. Bringing the patient self-determination act into practice. Nurs Manage 1991;22:29–32.

8. Jezewski MA, Finnell DS. The meaning of DNR status: oncology nurses' experiences with patients and families. Cancer Nurs 1998;21:212–21.

9. Johns JL. Advance directives and opportunities for nurses. Image J Nurs Sch 1996;28:149–53.

10. Mezey M, Evans LK, Golub ZD. The patient self-determination act: sources of concern for nurses. Nurs Outlook 1994;42:30–8.

11. Forbes S, Bern-Klug M, Gessert C. End-of-life decision making for nursing home residents with dementia. Image J Nurs Sch 2000;32:251–8.

12. Levy CR, Ely EW, Payne K, et al. Quality of dying and death in two medical ICUs: Perceptions of family and clinicians. Chest 2005;127:1775–83.

13. Rushton CH, Spencer KL, Johanson WN. Bringing end-of-life care out of the shadows. Holist Nurs Pract 2004;18:313–7.

14. Wilkie DJ, Judge MK, Wells MJ, et al. Excellence in teaching end-of-life care: a new multimedia toolkit for nurse educators. Nurs Health Care Perspect 2001; 22:226–30.

15. Approaching Death: Improving Care at the End of Life. Available at: http://books.nap.edu/catalog/5801.html. Accessed August 10, 2009.

16. Describing death in America. Accessed August 10, 2009 at http://books.nap.edu/html/describing_death/reportbrief.pdf.

17. The SUPPORT Principal Investigators. A controlled trial to improve care for seriously ill hospitalized patients. JAMA 1995;274:1591–8.

18. American Nurses Association. Compendium of position statements on the nurse's role in end-of-life decisions. Washington, DC: American Nurses Publishing; 1992.

19. Sherman DW, Matzo ML, Pitorak E, et al. Preparation and care at the time of death. J Nurses Staff Dev 2005;21:93–100.

20. National Hospice Foundation (n.d.). History of Hospice Care. Hospice: A historical perspective. Available at: http://www.nhpco.org/i4a/page/index.cfm?pageid=3285. Accessed June 25, 2007.

21. Kvale EA, Williams BR, Bolden JL, et al. The balm of Gilead project: a demonstration project on end-of-life care for safety-net populations. J Palliat Med 2004;7:486–93.

22. Musgrave CF, Allen CE, Allen GJ. Spirituality and health for women of color. Am J Public Health 2002;94:557–60.

23. Taylor EJ. Spiritual needs of patients with cancer and family caregivers. Cancer Nurs 2003;26:260–6.

24. Shrank WH, Kutner JS, Richardson T, et al. Focus group findings about the influence of culture on communication preferences in end-of-life care. J Gen Intern Med 2005;20:703–9.

25. Sullivan MA, Muskin PR, Feldman SJ, et al. Effects of religiosity on patients' perceptions of do-not-resuscitate status. Psychosomatics 2005;45:119–28.

26. Robinson R. End-of-life education in the undergraduate nursing curricula. Dimens Crit Care Nurs 2004;23:89–92.

27. Bjarnason D. Concept analysis of religiosity. Home Health Care Manag Pract 2007;19:350–5.

28. Ang D, Ibrahim SA, Burant CJ, et al. Ethnic differences in the perception of prayer and consideration of joint arthroplasty. Med Care 2002;40:471–6.

29. Kendler KS, Gardner CO, Prescott CA. Religion, psychopathology, and substance use and abuse: a multimeasure, genetic-epidemiologic study. Am J Psychiatry 1997;154:322–9.

30. Kendler KS, Liu XQ, Gardner CO, et al. Dimensions of religiosity and their relationship to lifetime psychiatric and substance use disorders. Am J Psychiatry 2003;160:496–503.

31. Oyama O, Koenig HG. Religious beliefs and practices in family medicine. Arch Fam Med 1998;7:431–5.
32. Steffen PR, Hinderliter AL, Blumenthal JA, et al. Religious coping, ethnicity, and ambulatory blood pressure. Psychosom Med 2001;63:523–30.
33. Foster D. Religion and medicine: the physician's perspective. In: Marty ME, Vaux KL, editors. Health/medicine and the faith traditions. Philadelphia: Fortress Press; 1982. p. 245–70.
34. Hilton SC, Fellingham GW, Lyon JL. Suicide rates and religious commitment in young adult males in Utah. Am J Epidemiol 2002;155:413–9.
35. Miller L, Warner V, Wickramararatne P, et al. Religiosity and depression: ten-year follow-up of depressed mothers and offspring. J Am Acad Child Adolesc Psychiatry 1997;36:1416–25.
36. Miller L, Davies M, Greenwald S. Religiosity and substance use and abuse among adolescents in the national comorbidity survey. J Am Acad Child Adolesc Psychiatry 2000;39:1190–7.
37. Horowitz JL, Garber J. Relation of intelligence and religiosity to depressive disorders in offspring of depressed and nondepressed mothers. J Am Acad Child Adolesc Psychiatry 2003;42:578–86.
38. Miller L, Gur MMS. Religiosity, depression, and physical maturation in adolescent girls. J Am Acad Child Adolesc Psychiatry 2002;41:206–14.
39. Curlin FA, Roach CJ, Gorawara-Bhat R, et al. When patients choose faith over medicine: physician perspectives on religiously related conflict in the medical encounter. Arch Intern Med 2005;165:88–91.
40. Hickey KS, Lyckholm L. Child welfare versus parental autonomy: medical ethics, the law, and faith-based healing. Theor Med 2004;25:265–76.
41. The Florence Nightingale Pledge. 1893. Available at: http://www.nursingworld.org/FunctionalMenuCategories/AboutANA/WhereWeComeFrom_1/FlorenceNightingalePledge.aspx. Accessed June 7, 2009.
42. Baldacchino D, Draper P. Spiritual coping strategies: A review of the nursing literature. J Adv Nurs 2001;34:833–41.
43. Theis SL, Biordi DL, Coeling H, et al. Spirituality in caregiving and care receiving. Holist Nurs Pract 2003;17:48–55.
44. Curlin FA, Chin MH, Sellergren SA, et al. The association of physicians' religious characteristics with their attitudes and self-reported behaviors regarding religion and spirituality in the clinical encounter. Med Care 2006;44:446–53.
45. Smith LC, Friedman S, Nevid J. Clinical and sociocultural differences in African American and European American patients with panic disorder and agoraphobia. J Nerv Ment Dis 1999;187:549–60.
46. Curlin FA, Lawrence RE, Chin MJ, et al. Religion, conscience, and controversial clinical practices. N Engl J Med 2007;356:593–600.
47. Luckhaupt SE, Yi MS, Mueller CV, et al. Beliefs of primary care residents regarding spirituality and religion in clinical encounters with patients: a study at a Midwestern U.S. teaching institution. Acad Med 2005;80:560–70.
48. Wenger NS, Carmel S. Physicians' religiosity and end-of-life care attitudes and behaviors. Mt Sinai J Med 2004;71:335–43.
49. Wright KB. Professional, ethical, and legal implications for spiritual care in nursing. Image J Nurs Sch 1998;30(1):81–3.
50. Warner C. A tool for spiritual assessment and intervention. Top Emerg Med 2005; 27:186–91.

# Index

*Note:* Page numbers of article titles are in **boldface** type.

doi:10.1016/S0029-6465(09)00077-2
0029-6465/09/$ – see front matter

**United States Postal Service**

## Statement of Ownership, Management, and Circulation
### (All Periodicals Publications Except Requestor Publications)

| 1. Publication Title | 2. Publication Number | | | | | | | | 3. Filing Date |
|---|---|---|---|---|---|---|---|---|---|
| Nursing Clinics of North America | 5 | 9 | 8 | - | 9 | 9 | 6 | 0 | 9/15/09 |

| 4. Issue Frequency | 5. Number of Issues Published Annually | 6. Annual Subscription Price |
|---|---|---|
| Mar, Jun, Sep, Dec | 4 | $133.00 |

7. Complete Mailing Address of Known Office of Publication (Not printer) (Street, city, county, state, and ZIP+4®)

Elsevier Inc.
360 Park Avenue South
New York, NY 10010-1710

Contact Person: Stephen Bushing

Telephone (Include area code): 215-239-3688

8. Complete Mailing Address of Headquarters or General Business Office of Publisher (Not printer)

Elsevier Inc., 360 Park Avenue South, New York, NY 10010-1710

9. Full Names and Complete Mailing Addresses of Publisher, Editor, and Managing Editor (Do not leave blank)

Publisher (Name and complete mailing address)

John Schrefer, Elsevier, Inc., 1600 John F. Kennedy Blvd. Suite 1800, Philadelphia, PA 19103-2899

Editor (Name and complete mailing address)

Katie Hartner, Elsevier, Inc., 1600 John F. Kennedy Blvd. Suite 1800, Philadelphia, PA 19103-2899

Managing Editor (Name and complete mailing address)

Catherine Bewick, Elsevier, Inc., 1600 John F. Kennedy Blvd. Suite 1800, Philadelphia, PA 19103-2899

10. Owner (Do not leave blank. If the publication is owned by a corporation, give the name and address of the corporation immediately followed by the names and addresses of all stockholders owning or holding 1 percent or more of the total amount of stock. If not owned by a corporation, give the names and addresses of the individual owners. If owned by a partnership or other unincorporated firm, give its name and address as well as those of each individual owner. If the publication is published by a nonprofit organization, give its name and address.)

| Full Name | Complete Mailing Address |
|---|---|
| Wholly owned subsidiary of | 4520 East-West Highway |
| Reed/Elsevier, US holdings | Bethesda, MD 20814 |

11. Known Bondholders, Mortgagees, and Other Security Holders Owning or Holding 1 Percent or More of Total Amount of Bonds, Mortgages, or Other Securities. If none, check box.  ☐ None

| Full Name | Complete Mailing Address |
|---|---|
| N/A | |

12. Tax Status (For completion by nonprofit organizations authorized to mail at nonprofit rates) (Check one)
The purpose, function, and nonprofit status of this organization and the exempt status for federal income tax purposes:
☐ Has Not Changed During Preceding 12 Months
☐ Has Changed During Preceding 12 Months (Publisher must submit explanation of change with this statement)

PS Form 3526, September 2007 (Page 1 of 3 (Instructions Page 3)) PSN 7530-01-000-9931 PRIVACY NOTICE: See our Privacy policy in www.usps.com

---

| 13. Publication Title | 14. Issue Date for Circulation Data Below |
|---|---|
| Nursing Clinics of North America | September 2009 |

| 15. Extent and Nature of Circulation | | | Average No. Copies Each Issue During Preceding 12 Months | No. Copies of Single Issue Published Nearest to Filing Date |
|---|---|---|---|---|
| a. Total Number of Copies (Net press run) | | | 2950 | 2800 |
| b. Paid Circulation (By Mail and Outside the Mail) | (1) | Mailed Outside-County Paid Subscriptions Stated on PS Form 3541. (Include paid distribution above nominal rate, advertiser's proof copies, and exchange copies) | 1821 | 1597 |
| | (2) | Mailed In-County Paid Subscriptions Stated on PS Form 3541 (Include paid distribution above nominal rate, advertiser's proof copies, and exchange copies) | | |
| | (3) | Paid Distribution Outside the Mails Including Sales Through Dealers and Carriers, Street Vendors, Counter Sales, and Other Paid Distribution Outside USPS® | 476 | 490 |
| | (4) | Paid Distribution by Other Classes Mailed Through the USPS (e.g. First-Class Mail®) | | |
| c. Total Paid Distribution (Sum of 15b (1), (2), (3), and (4)) | | ▲ | 2297 | 2187 |
| d. Free or Nominal Rate Distribution (By Mail and Outside the Mail) | (1) | Free or Nominal Rate Outside-County Copies Included on PS Form 3541 | 76 | 73 |
| | (2) | Free or Nominal Rate In-County Copies Included on PS Form 3541 | | |
| | (3) | Free or Nominal Rate Copies Mailed at Other Classes Through the USPS (e.g. First-Class Mail) | | |
| | (4) | Free or Nominal Rate Distribution Outside the Mail (Carriers or other means) | | |
| e. Total Free or Nominal Rate Distribution (Sum of 15d (1), (2), (3) and (4)) | | ▲ | 76 | 73 |
| f. Total Distribution (Sum of 15c and 15e) | | ▲ | 2373 | 2260 |
| g. Copies not Distributed (See instructions to publishers #4 (page #3)) | | ▲ | 577 | 540 |
| h. Total (Sum of 15f and g) | | ▲ | 2950 | 2800 |
| i. Percent Paid (15c divided by 15f times 100) | | | 96.80% | 96.77% |

16. Publication of Statement of Ownership

☐ If the publication is a general publication, publication of this statement is required. Will be printed in the December 2009 issue of this publication.  ☐ Publication not required

17. Signature and Title of Editor, Publisher, Business Manager, or Owner

*Stephen R. Bushing* — Subscription Services Coordinator

Date: September 15, 2009

I certify that all information furnished on this form is true and complete. I understand that anyone who furnishes false or misleading information on this form or who omits material or information requested on the form may be subject to criminal sanctions (including fines and imprisonment) and/or civil sanctions (including civil penalties).

PS Form 3526, September 200 (Page 2 of 3)

# Moving?

## Make sure your subscription moves with you!

To notify us of your new address, find your **Clinics Account Number** (located on your mailing label above your name), and contact customer service at:

Email: **journalscustomerservice-usa@elsevier.com**

**800-654-2452** (subscribers in the U.S. & Canada)
**314-447-8871** (subscribers outside of the U.S. & Canada)

Fax number: **314-447-8029**

**Elsevier Health Sciences Division**
**Subscription Customer Service**
**3251 Riverport Lane**
**Maryland Heights, MO 63043**